How to Get Rid of Your Skinny Self

Through

High Intensity Training

By

Edgar G. Garcia

Dedication:

I would like to dedicate this book to my beautiful loving wife, *Shiela H. Garcia* and to my very supportive and loving parents, *Rodolfo* and *Normita Garcia*.

Thank You:

I would like to thank the following people who contributed to this book:

Shiela Garcia

Jarrod Bryant

Jaime Augusto Barriento Jr. (for doing home gym training)

Kyle Babb

Author Salas

Jorge Coky Sanchez

…and thank you to Steve Spreyer for the Classic Physique Tank Top that I wore in some of the pictures. Also thank you to Denny and Diana Kakos for letting us use their gym.

I would like to say a special thank you to my beautiful loving late wife, *Adriana Garcia*, who suggested I write this book and for her tremendous contribution.

Please Note:

Engaging in any strenuous physical activities and following any dietary recommendation runs a certain risk that can potentially result in a physical injury or even death. The author of this book is not responsible in the decision that the readers have made in following his guidelines. Always consult with your physician before following any strenuous physical activities and any dietary recommendation.

TABLE OF CONTENT

INTRODUCTION

I remember the day I was at the auto parts store in Corona, California. It was a very warm day in 2007. I was wearing a white t-shirt along with my favorite camouflage shorts. I was hot, sweaty, and dirty from fixing my brother Edwin's '89 Firebird. I was in line to make a purchase and there were several customers ahead of me. Over the counter there was this thin auto parts clerk perhaps in his early 30's that was ringing us up. He kept eyeing me up and down for some reason. I thought he was eyeing me because I was sweaty and dirty. It made me feel uncomfortable for a moment.

When it was my turn to be rang up he asked me, "You lift weights?" I said yes. Then he asked me, "Hey, what do you recommend so I could gain some weight and get rid of my skinny self?" I recommended a couple of things to him when it comes to weight training and eating. I wanted to go more into details with him but I couldn't because there were other people waiting in line. He knew it as well. So after he rang me up we parted.

After I finished working on my brother's car I went home and thought about that clerk from the auto parts store. I pulled out some of my old pictures where I was very thin. My late wife, Adriana, took notice and asked me why I was looking at my past pictures. I told her about him and how I remember being painfully thin myself. I told her he wasn't the first one to ask me about gaining weight and developing their muscles. I've been asked several times before at the gym, at school, at my former websites, and at work. I told Adriana the process I went through back then and how I was able to get rid of my skinny self. She then said to me, "You know mijo, you should write a book about it and title it, 'How to Get Rid of Your Skinny Self.'" After she said that she giggled.

It was February 14th, 1989 - Valentine's Day. To most people this was a celebration of love with their significant other or perhaps discovering what love is by asking someone out for a date. To me it was very different. I discovered love on this day, but it wasn't with a girl. I found love that day by joining Mt. Olympus Gym in Corona, California. I was a shy and very thin 18 year old teenager who made a big leap by signing up for a gym membership. I was going beyond my comfort zone from the little bedroom that my brother, Edwin, and I shared where I had my tiny plastic plated cement filled weights and vinyl covered bench were set. My goal was one thing and one thing only, to get rid of my skinny self.

My family and I moved to Corona, California from Tustin in the fall of 1988. I was a senior at Corona Senior High School and I was a part-time worker for McDonald's fast food restaurant. After school I made my way to work in my ten speed bike. I would always pass by this gym, Mt. Olympus Gym. Several times I would look through its windows and watch the men and some women working out with weights and machines. To me they all looked very muscular and very strong. I could hear them grunting and I could see their sweat covered skin glistening under the fluorescent lights above them. I was very much intimidated to go inside and have a closer look.

After looking through the gym's windows for several months I finally mustard enough courage to go inside and inquire about a membership. The gym looked totally different from the inside than from the outside. The people who were working out looked even bigger. The grunting sound was louder and the energy coming from them was off the wall! There was a strong musky smell of sweat and un-deodorized armpits in the air.

The gym reminded me so much of the pictures I've seen in the old muscle magazines I had. It was like stepping into the *pumping iron* era where big muscular guys like Arnold Schwarzenegger, Lou Ferrigno, Franco Columbo, Ed Corney, Ken Waller, and other top bodybuilding champs from way back then used to train, because the exercise equipments were so similar to that time and it had that feel to it.

I went to the reception desk and I was met by this tall six foot three, burly, heavily muscled Greek man by the name of Denny Kakos. He was the owner of Mt. Olympus Gym. He later on became the CEO and president of INBA, PNBA, and ABA organization, the largest natural and drugfree bodybuilding association in the west coast. I remember him taking my $29.95 initiation fee along with my $14.95 monthly dues. He then went to his file cabinet and took out a chart that showed a diagram of the human anatomy and a measuring tape. He told me he liked taking stats of all his members. With a chart on his hand he asked me to stand on the weight scale. I clearly remember tipping the weight scale at 118lbs. He then used his measuring tape and asked me to flex my bicep. It came out to be 11 ¾ inches. He then measured my chest which was 29 inches and then my waistline which was 26 inches. He went on and measured my other body parts.

"So do I have a chance of becoming Mr. Universe someday?" I asked him with a smile.

He had a serious look on his face. His big bright green eyes began probing me from head to toe and from side to side. I was waiting for him to tell me about the rigors of training, the heavy lifting I have to put my body through, the hours I have to spend in the gym and how in the end I would be rewarded with a big muscular body. But the first thing Denny said to me, "You have to eat."

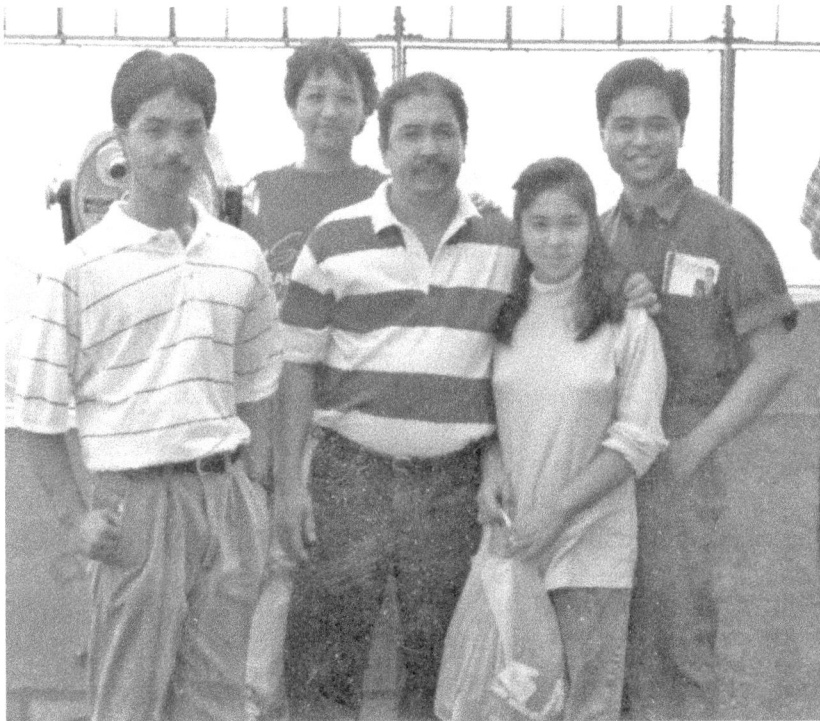

Me at the left with my family:
My mom, Normita, my dad, Rodolfo, my sister, Elaine,
and my brother, Edwin.

There are a number of men out there as well as women who feel the same way as I did back then when it comes to being too thin. Nobody wants to look like a stick figure, look sickly, or look like a malnourished individual. Growing up as a teenager and into early adulthood I've never learned to cope with my thin look. This sort of thing runs in both sides of my family. Where the men are thin at first and then they eventually develop a pudgy looking belly as they get older, while still retaining their skinny arms and legs. I wanted so bad to do something about it.

When I was a kid I grew up admiring muscular men like Lou Ferrigno in the Incredible Hulk TV series, Steve Reeves in Hercules movies, Charles Atlas who turned his skinny body into a strong and muscular one. I knew early on in my life that I wanted to be like them, strong and well built. So I embarked on a muscle building quest.

As you can see by the title itself that this book caters to people who suffered from being naturally too thin. The goal of this book is not to turn you into a world class Mr. Universe or Mrs. Universe type physique, but to help you achieve a muscular built that will help you get rid of your skinny self.

Yes my friend, you will be going through what is called bodybuilding. Please don't be intimidated by the word, bodybuilding. Most people automatically conjured in their mind of heavily muscled men and women who goes up on stage in their tight spandex or bikinis and pose in front of a large audience.

The word bodybuilding means just that, building your body. For the sake of this book it means building your body in order to get rid of your skinny self. You'll be using weights, nutrition, and recuperation in order to achieve this.

The book will go through what I call the Trinity of Bodybuilding: Training, Nutrition, and Recuperation. These are the three most important components in bodybuilding. This book will go through each one so that you can have an in-depth understanding of it and how it will help you in your progress. First we will go through some subcomponents that you should know and have such as the importance of keeping a training log, setting long term and short term goals, understanding training principles, and other necessities.

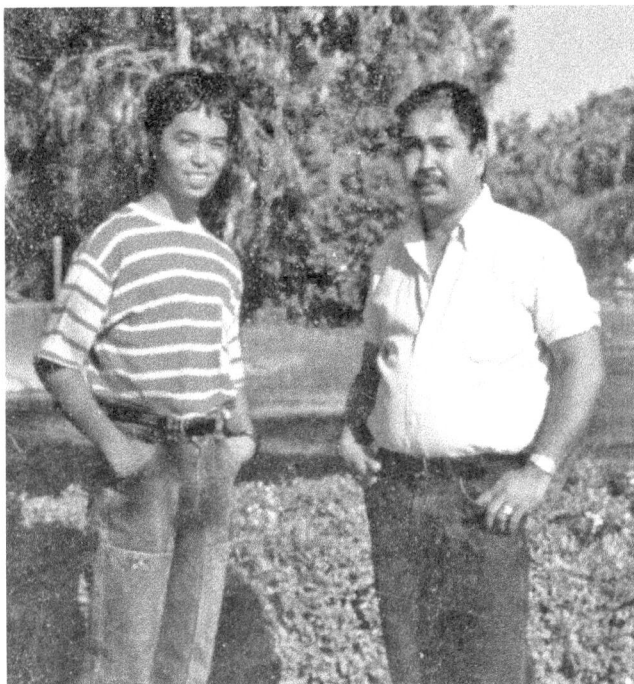

My dad was 160lbs in this picture while I was 118lbs.

"If my mind can conceive it, and my heart can believe it – then I can achieve it."

--- Muhammad Ali

PART ONE

Where to Start

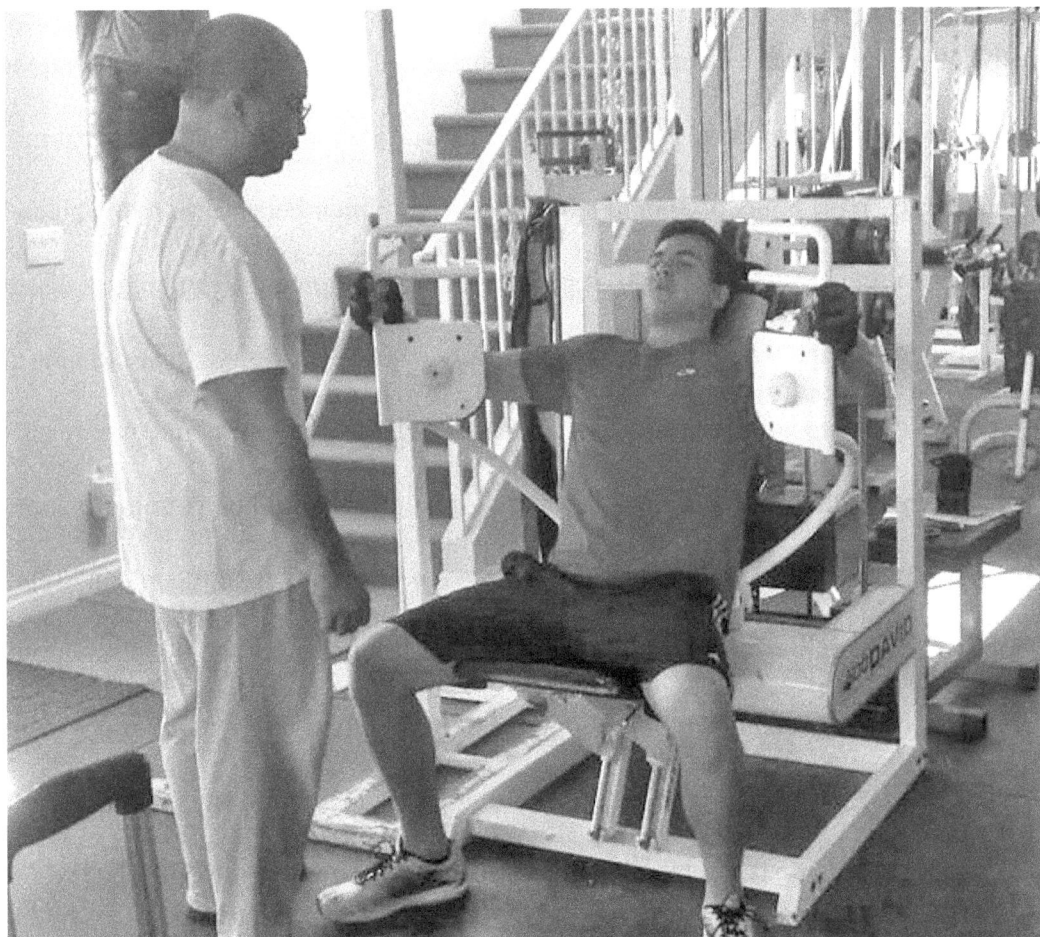

With Arthur Salas

CHAPTER 1

FINDING A GYM

So if you have finally decided that you want to get rid of that skinny look of yours then I say to you, "Congratulation." You've just taken a major step in your life. You want muscles and the good health that comes along with it. Now that you've made that decision you still need to make another decision, where to train.

There are only two places you can train, either at home or at the gym. There are advantages and disadvantages to them. If you decide to train at home then the major advantage here is that you can train at anytime. You don't have to worry about the gym's closing and opening hours. You don't have to worry about the rush hours that most gyms have between the hours of 3pm to 8pm. Where gym members are wall to wall and you end up waiting for them to finish using the exercise equipment. The biggest disadvantage to training at home would be the lack of variety in your exercises. It would take quite a bit of investing in good exercise equipments in order to get your home gym ready for your bodybuilding ambition. Another big disadvantage would be your motivation. This is more true for extroverted people. They need to be around other people in order to feel motivated. People who are introverted, like myself, have no problems being motivated.

The old fashion pumping iron gyms like Mt. Olympus Gym are pretty much gone. This type of gym was where heavily muscular men and women tend to conjugate. You can actually see sweat and blood come off them-well maybe not blood. Today's gyms or fitness centers, as they are called, are corporately owned. It's a multi-billion dollar business where the small pumping iron like gyms can't compete. Of course there is nothing wrong with corporate gyms. Many of them tend to have more and better exercise equipments than the old fashion pumping iron like gyms. But the energy, motivation, and especially the camaraderie in pumping iron like gyms are often times way better than any corporate gyms.

If you have decided to train in the gym then I suggest you open up your phonebook and see what gyms or fitness centers are in your area. Set up an appointment to meet with a representative. Visit the gym at its busiest hours which is usually between the hours of 3pm to 8pm during weekdays. So you can see just how crowded the gym can get. Ask the rep what the hours are when the gym is the least crowded and plan on visiting again at those hours. Be sure to visit all the gyms in your area before making a final decision. See who has the best equipments and the best price.

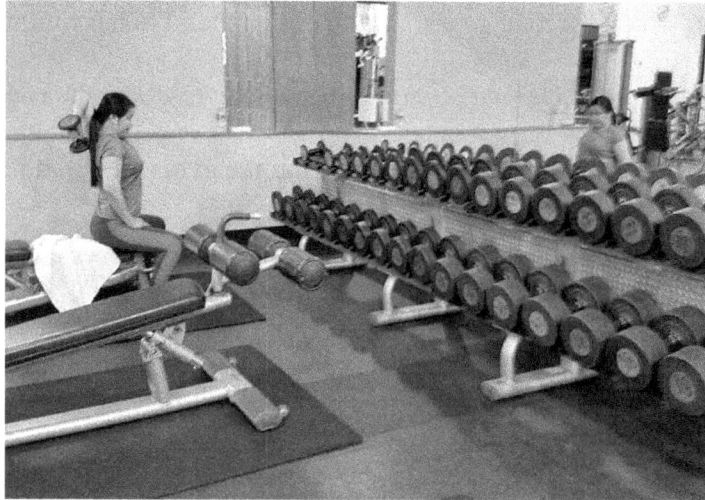

Shiela Garcia working out at a corporate gym.

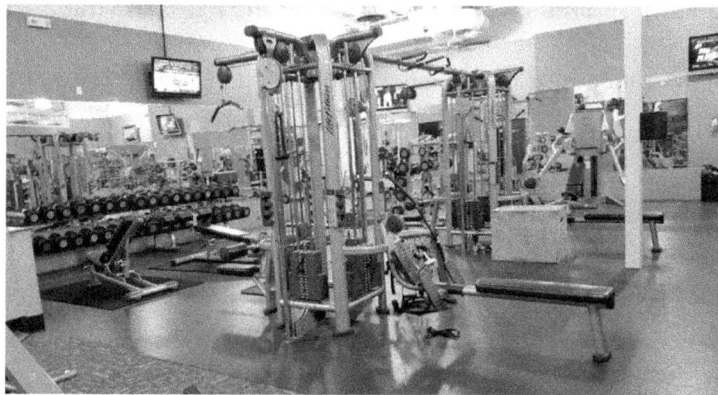

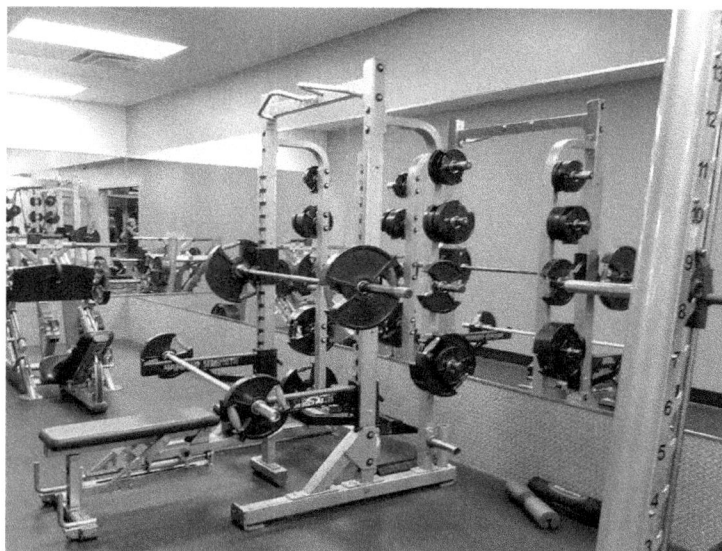

CHAPTER 2

WHAT YOU NEED FOR YOUR WORKOUT

Now that you've joined a gym or got all your home gym equipments set you are now ready to workout. But there are things you still need before you dive into it.

Workout Attire

I recommend you wear clothes that you feel comfortable sweating in. For me I've always preferred wearing a tank top, cotton made shorts, thick padded socks, and a pair of worn out sneakers(so I can do calf raises properly). I don't recommend you wear heavy sweats unless you live in a very cold climate.

It is very important to allow heat from your body to expel during workouts in order to allow your body to cool off. Wearing the least amount of clothes will help do so. Heavy clothes will only keep the heat in your body instead of allowing it to circulate out. If not you may find yourself feeling drain of energy from your uncirculated body heat.

Weight Training Belt

I recommend you have this handy when you do exercises such as squats and leg presses. This will help keep your lower back and abs steady. Other than that you don't really need to wear them, unless if you are like me with a bad lower back. In that case wear it at all times.

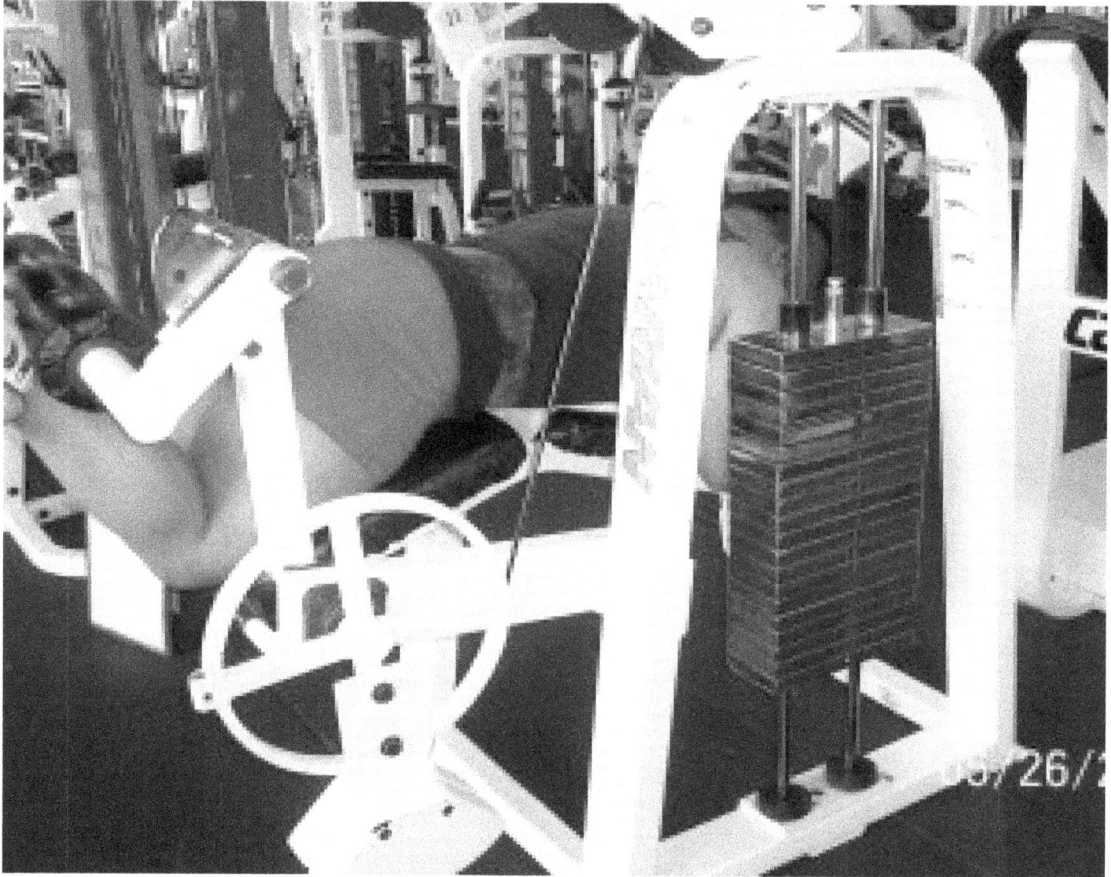

Weight Training Belt helps me with my lower back pain.

Wrist/Grip Straps

This comes in handy later on as you progressively get stronger and stronger in your pulling exercises for your back and shoulders. For example, if you are doing wide pulldowns for your back, the strength of your back will exceed the strength of your grip. When that happens you wouldn't be able to properly complete your set. Wrist/grip straps will help ensure that your grip doesn't fail before your back does. Keep in mind though that you should only use wrist/grip straps when you need too. Using it to do all your exercises will not help develop the strength of your grip.

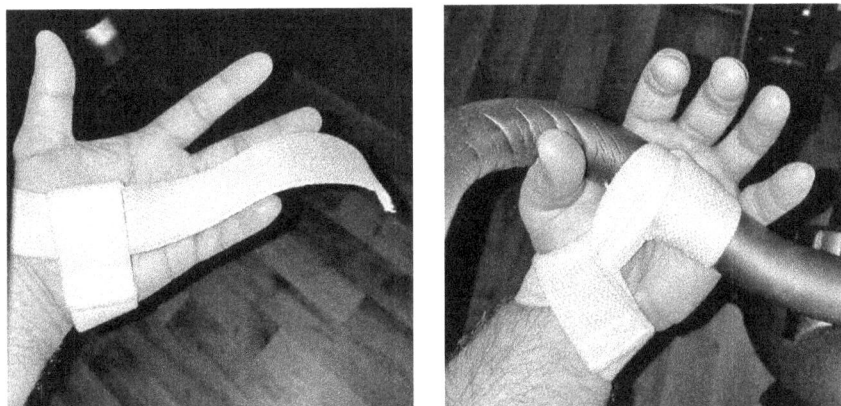

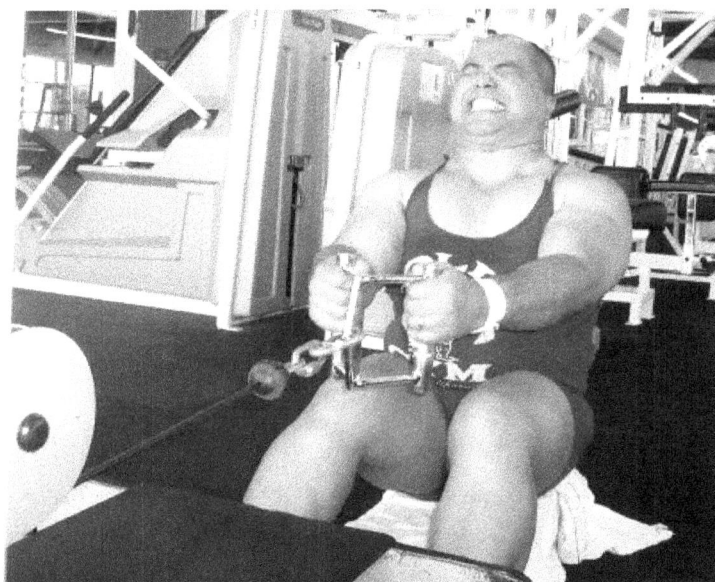

Wrist/Grip Straps help me grip this 300lbs weight on Seated Rows.

Water Bottle

This is a must have during your workouts. If you are training hard, breathing hard, and sweating hard then you are losing water. Having a water bottle close to you and taking constant sips from it will help replenish some of the water you lost during the process of exercise. Water also helps in keeping your body to stay cool.

Towel

Towel is used not only to wipe your sweat, but also for sanitary reasons. You should drape it over the exercise equipment that you are using. The reason for draping the towel over the exercise equipment is because a number of gym members have used it before you and they've left behind their residue of sweat and moisture from their bodies. These are magnets for germs and bacteria.

I remember my first couple of years training in the gym. I've developed all sorts of skin rashes on my upper back, because I wore tank tops when I workout. The doctor asked me if I had been using a towel to drape over the exercise equipment. I told him no. He told me to start doing that.

Remember too to wash your hands after you are through exercising.

Training Log

This is another must have! This is something that you must take with you every time you go to the gym. A training log is where you have written down some of the exercises you will be doing, the amount of weights you plan on using, and how many reps you are shooting for. You must jot down what your goals are on that day and how you plan on accomplishing it. A training log doesn't have to be fancy. It can be just a piece of paper kept on a notebook, or a binder.

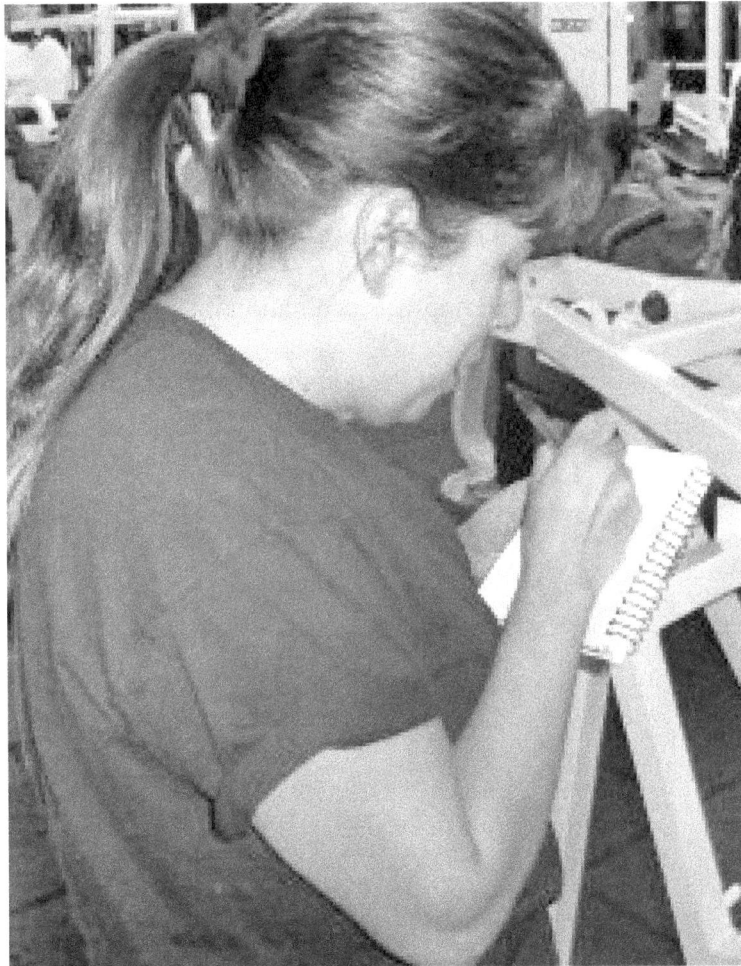

Here Adriana Garcia is writing down the number of reps she did after the exercise.

CHAPTER 3

IMPORTANCE OF SETTING YOUR GOALS

I remember when I first stepped in to Mt. Olympus Gym at age 18 and weighing in at 118lbs, I thought to myself back then how I wanted to be the strongest, biggest, and baddest guy in the gym. And I thought back then training 6 days a week for 2 to 3 hours a day would help me reach my goal. Well it didn't happen in one year or even in two years, but my goal back then was to enter a teen natural bodybuilding contest before I turn 20.

Just 9 days shy of my 20th birthday I decided to enter a teen natural bodybuilding contest in my area. Just to try it out, plus I wanted to see how well I would do. Little did I know that the contest I was entering was at a national level where I competed against other teenagers from different parts of the country. I was competing against teenagers who were from Arizona, Michigan, Texas and so forth. I came in dead last.

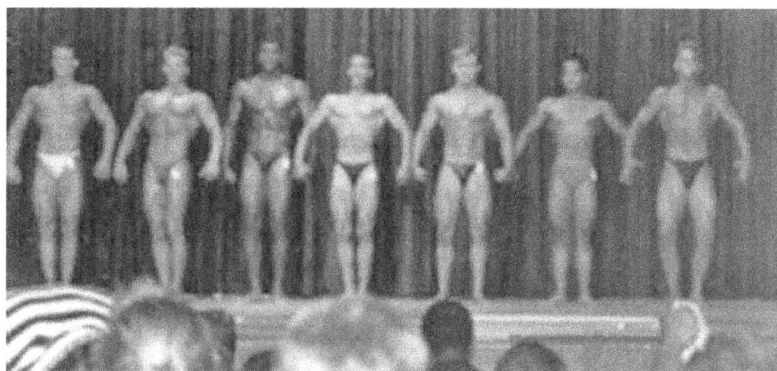

I'm the 2nd one to the right. The winner was the second one to the left from Arizona. I was small and thin looking compare to them.

After that contest I knew that I needed to make more gains. I still had that thin look. I still trained 6 days a week for 2 to 3 hours at a time. I very much did this during my early 20's. I also ate whatever was on the table, but still I couldn't get rid of my skinny look. I've given up on training and on my goals all together and paid more attention to my other favorite hobby, which was cycling.

I remember not going to the gym anymore for a couple of months. During those couple months was when my body went into a rest mode. I was burned out from weight training. I did nothing for a couple of months other than ride my bike, go to work, go to college and sleep all day long. My body was becoming what it was before. Whatever muscles I gained I was losing it and I looked even more thin.

I didn't like it. I needed to go back to the gym and start working out again. I wanted so bad to get rid of my skinny self. When I went back and started training again I just didn't have that same drive anymore. My energy and motivation wasn't all there. So I stopped going again.

My day of epiphany came to me when I went to the local public library and found a used book on sale for a dime. It was titled "The Nautilus Book," written by Dr. Ellington Darden. It was from this book that I learned what frequency and duration means and why too much weight training is not productive. Dr. Darden called this *overtraining*. A word I have never heard before, or even read from my vast collection of bodybuilding books and magazines.

With me doing 6 days a week workout for 2 to 3 hours at a time proved that I was indeed overtraining. I never gave my body a chance to recuperate in order for it to grow in strength and size. I will discuss this more in details.

I bought more books written by Ellington Darden I discovered another word that he often talked about, *H.I.T.,* short for *High Intensity Training.* He mentioned in order for muscles to grow the intensity of weight training must be high. Again, I will discuss this more in details as well.

I remember getting a piece of paper and writing down what I needed to do. This would be the start of my training log. When I went back to the gym it felt like I was stepping in the gym for the first time again. I have a new found knowledge and a better sense of understanding in how to approach my training. Once I got into applying this new found knowledge I was on a path to progress. The skinny look I once had was slowly disappearing. My arms, legs, chest, back, and so on were getting thicker.

Since I was making excellent progress, I needed to set my goals. I had a short term goal and that was to break into 160lbs, the same weight as my dad. Since I weighted 127lbs at the time I thought that was achievable. Sure enough I did break it and not only did I break it, I actually did better than what I expected. I actually got to 170lbs. I kept setting up short term goals like that till eventually I got to my long term goal, which was to weigh 200lbs. It took me several years to achieve this and boy was it worth it.

(BODY MEASUREMENT & GOAL)

LOST BODY FAT

DATE:	12-12-86	DATE:	10-2-87	DATE:	4-21-88	
WEIGHT:	—	WEIGHT:	—	WEIGHT:	127 lbs	
HEIGHT:	5'7"	HEIGHT:	5'7"	HEIGHT:	5'7"	
NECK:	—	NECK:	14⅜	NECK:	—	
CHEST:	36½	CHEST:	36¹³⁄₁₆	CHEST:	—	
UPPER ARM:	13⅛	UPPER ARM:	12⅛	UPPER ARM:	12½	
LOWER ARM:	—	LOWER ARM:	10½	LOWER ARM:	—	
WAIST:	28½	WAIST:	—	WAIST:	—	
THIGH UPPER:	—	THIGH UPPER:	—	THIGH UPPER:	—	
THIGH LOWER:	—	THIGH LOWER:	—	THIGH LOWER:	—	
CALF:	—	CALF:	14⅞"	CALF:	15"	

DATE:	2-15-89	DATE:	8-26-89	DATE:	2-19-90	
WEIGHT:	141½ lbs	WEIGHT:	157 lbs	WEIGHT:	153 lbs	
NECK:	14½"	NECK:	15⅛"	NECK:	16"	
CHEST:	37"	CHEST:	40½"	CHEST:	41"	
UPPER ARM:	12¾"	UPPER ARM:	14½	UPPER ARM:	14½"	
LOWER ARM:	11"	LOWER ARM:	12	LOWER ARM:	12"	
WAIST:	28½	WAIST:	31½"	WAIST:	31"	
UPPER THIGH:	21"	UPPER THIGH:	23"	UPPER THIGH:	23"	
LOWER THIGH:	—	LOWER THIGH:	20"	LOWER THIGH:	20"	
CALF:	—	CALF:	15½"	CALF:	16"	

GOAL TO PASS

WEIGHT:	170 lbs	2-91		UPPER THIGH:	25	3-27-91	30"
NECK:	17"	5-13-91		LOWER THIGH:	22"	3-27-91	28
CHEST:	45"	4-91 50"		CALF:	17"	5-13-91	26
UPPER ARM:	16	2-91 20					
LOWER ARM:	14"	been better N.A.					
WAIST:	30"	Must maintain					

I copied Denny Kakos' stat sheet and wrote my own. I wrote the dates down once I broke that goal. This is perhaps something you want to do as well.

I wrote down my stats on a piece of paper because I was making excellent progress. I no longer had that skinny look anymore. My friends, families, and my buddies at the gym gave me positive feedback. I was no longer that skinny 118lbs weakling who kept looking through the windows of Mt. Olympus Gym from the outside. I've done it! I've reached my goal.

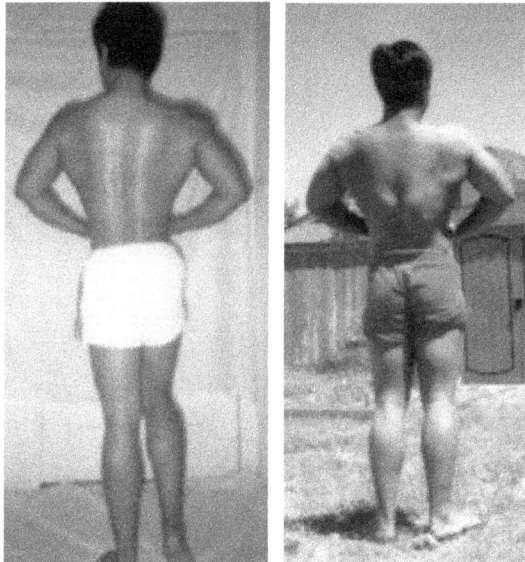

Here I went from 127lbs to 141lbs in less than 5 months.

In order for you to get rid of your skinny self you must have short term goals and long term goals. It makes training and your dedication all the more meaningful and rewarding. Be sure to be realistic with yourself and don't set goals that would seem impossible to achieve.

Let us say that you are 5'10" tall and you weigh about 150lbs. Your long term goal is to look like a buff 210lbs and you would like to achieve this in 4 years time. That is a very realistic goal to achieve. Now if you said 280lbs in one year then you have a problem. Unless you did nothing but stuff your face with donuts and pizza then yes you might be able to achieve 280lbs. That is, if you don't mind looking like a sumo wrestler.

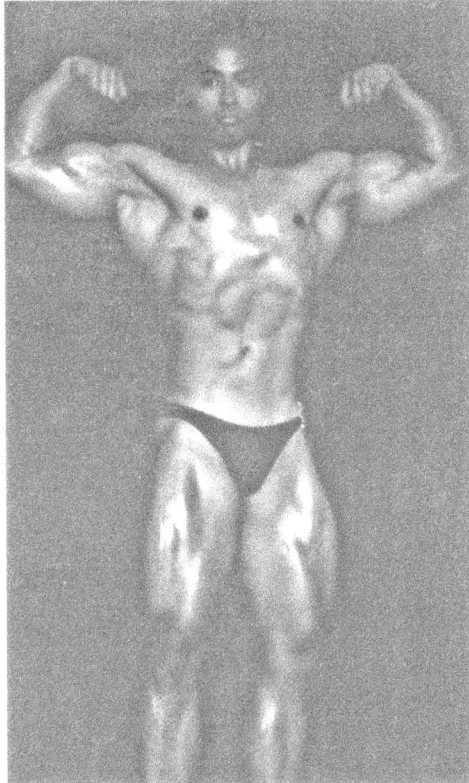

After a couple of years on H.I.T. I returned to compete in natural bodybuilding and took 3rd.

So if your goal is to go from 150lbs to 210lbs in 4 years and achieve it by way of mostly muscles then you must set up your short term goal for your first year. If you are a beginner and this is indeed your first year, it is alright to set your short term goal in gaining 20lbs. Then the next year set it at 15lbs. Set it again for 15lbs the year after that and another 10lbs the year after. This way in 4 years time you would have achieved your long term goal. Some of you may achieve this earlier and some of you may require more time. It really does depend on you and your genetics.

You may think that 20lbs, 15lbs, or 10lbs doesn't sound much, but have you ever bought freshly grounded beef at those weights? It's a lot of beef isn't it? Now imagine that in you and in 4 years time. You would have put on 60lbs of mostly muscles. Now that's something to look forward too. Just be patient!

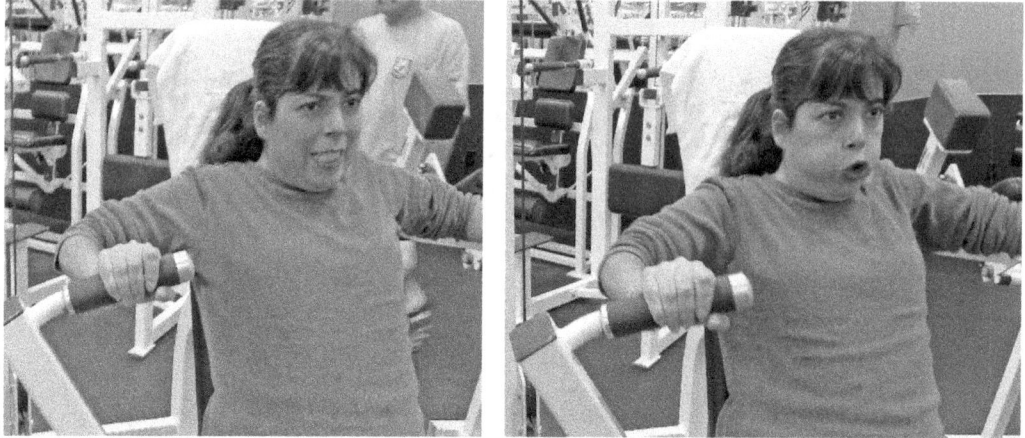

Adriana Garcia

Doing Machine Chest Press.

"Fear is a liar. The truth is you can, you must, you will.

So just do it."

-- Anonymous

PART II

The Trinity in Bodybuilding

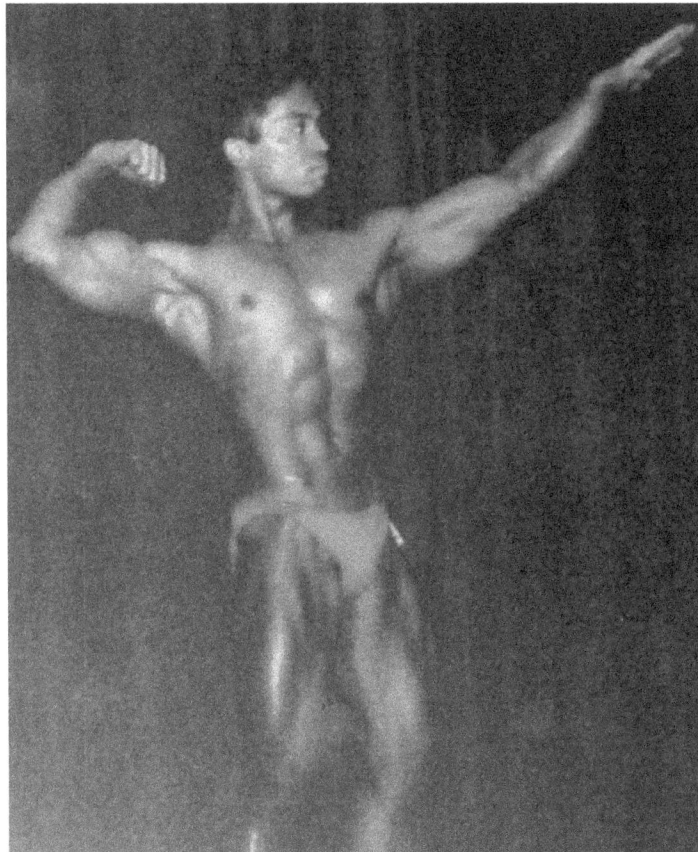

CHAPTER 4

HOW EXERCISES STIMULATE THE MUSCLES

(First Part in the Trinity)

The best way for you to get rid of your skinny self is to do weight training. You probably already know that. It's what led you into picking up my book. Weight training is indeed your key, along with proper nutrition, and recuperation.

Weight training is also referred to as resistance training. You'll see that I tend to bounce between these two terms. Weight training is nothing more than a bodybuilding process where your muscles go against an object that creates high level of resistance. The point of this is to create enough stress on your muscles that it forces them to adapt by getting stronger. As you get stronger the size of your muscles will eventually increase. This is your body's way of adapting from the stress which only weight training can provide.

Each muscle in your body is composed of millions of muscle fibers. They are covered by sheath like tissues and the ends of each muscle are connected to another tissue that is both tough and flexible, known as tendons. These tendons are connected to your bones. So when your muscles contract it moves the bones along with it. That is why this system is called musculoskeletal system. There are other types of muscles as well like the cardiac muscles of your heart or the smooth muscles found in your intestine, both are involuntary muscles. But for the most part we will only concern ourselves with the musculoskeletal system, which are voluntary.

Many of the things that you do in your daily life are in a form of resistance. Whether you are mowing the lawn, climbing up the stairs, or picking up a book off a shelf and so on those are all resistance activities-not necessarily resistance training. Such activities have very little or no affect whatsoever to cause your muscles to adapt by way of strength and size increase.

What's needed is for the resistance to be at a high level in order to cause the muscles to adapt by getting stronger and increasing in size. You can pick up a 5lb dumbbell and do 100 curls with it. If that 5lb is too easy there wouldn't be any cause or reason for your muscles to adapt. Now if you picked up a 50lb dumbbell and you struggled to even do 8 curls with it then you have given your body a reason to adapt.

H.I.T.

High Intensity Training, it is all about high levels of resistance imposed on your muscles. This is your key in stimulating the muscles to the fullest. Proper use of weight apparatus such as dumbbells, barbells, pulley machines, machines and such can provide this. For example, if you want your chest to increase in size or mass you can target that by doing bench press and dumbbell flys. You can't otherwise do this by pushing a lawnmower. The levels of resistance have to be so high that your chest muscles would be forced to get stronger and grow in size.

There is a catch to this. The higher you go on the level of resistance the shorter your workouts must become and less frequent. Therefore, the stronger and the bigger you get, the shorter the workout has to be and the more time you have to give your muscles to rest. I will explain this more when we get to recuperation. Just keep this in

31

mind, runners can never sprint a 26 mile marathon. It is physically impossible. Just like how most people can never do 100 curls with 50lb dumbbell, maybe a few can, but with 5lbs most definitely.

Originators of H.I.T.

Before I continue on discussing H.I.T., I need to give credit to those who pioneered it. The very first to create and advocate *High Intensity Training* was the late Author Jones. His former student, Dr. Ellington Darden, put his theory into perspective through his series of writings that resulted in a number of book publications spanning from the 1970's to today. You can find them in just about any bookstores. Dr. Darden also wrote a number of articles for fitness magazines.

I owe much gratitude to Dr. Darden for instilling the knowledge and wisdom in me on how to approach weight training. If it wasn't for him I would still be spending 2 to 3 hours working out in the gym. I would be going 5 to 6 times a week.

I also like to give credit to the late Mr. Universe, Mike Mentzer. Mike was one of my bodybuilding idols since my high school years. Since Mike and I were the height and body structure I admired him and wanted to look like him. Funny thing was, I didn't know Mike was also a student of Author Jones and a H.I.T. advocate. I've only looked at his pictures in muscle magazines and I never went beyond that. Back then I always thought training 6 days a week for 2 to 3 hours was the norm and I thought that was how Mike trained as well. It was indeed a bonus knowing my bodybuilding idol was a High Intensity Trainer. Mike also has a number of book publications that I highly recommend.

Applying H.I.T.

High Intensity Training or H.I.T. for short means going beyond your comfort zone. Yes, it is hard work. But it is a tolerable hard work. No, you are not going to be one of those people who weaseled their way through their workout by not pushing it hard and then pray that you would make some gains. No, that won't be you, because you will push it hard. Prayers won't be needed because it is guaranteed that you will make progress from this.

Here's an example of H.I.T. Let's say you picked up a barbell weighing 75lbs and you did 10 repetition curls with it and then you decided to stop and put it down. You just made a big mistake! You shouldn't have stopped your curls at the 10th rep. You should have kept going till you can't do one more, till you can no longer move the weight, not even by an inch. If you were to do it this way, then, that my friend, is what H.I.T. is all about. You went beyond your comfort zone. Rests assure you have stimulated your biceps muscles to their fullest.

Sorry if I disappointed you there with the words, "hard work." There really is no other way around of getting rid of your skinny self. But it is indeed brief and infrequent since H.I.T. is very demanding on the body. Your workouts may only take 20 minutes and at most 30 minutes in duration. And you only train twice a week. Again, I will explain this more as you continue to read.

Now this short and infrequent workout may appeal to a lot of you who are busybodies. It certainly did to me since back then I decided to go to school fulltime along with a full-time job. Whereas before training 6 days a week for 2 to 3 hours at a time it was almost impossible for me to go to school and work full-time. I had to work part-time and go to school part-time. Plus after this type of workout I barely had enough energy for anything. All I wanted to do was go home and go to sleep.

Some of you might get a little squeamish at the thought of doing *High Intensity Training.* Believe it or not to this day I still encounter people that are squeamish about it. Going beyond your comfort zone sounds too painful. I know that many of you who are painfully thin ended up this way because you've managed to avoid pushing your body hard, but if you really want to get rid of your skinny self this truly is the best way. At first the workout will feel sort of weird and uncomfortable, but in time your mind and body will learn to adapt. This adaptation is your key to success in getting rid of your skinny self.

What Exactly Does Intensity Mean?

When you hear the word intensity you may tend to conjure up a notion that one has to be able to bench press over 300lbs and to squat over 500lbs. Intensity is not all about how much weight you can lift. Rather it's relative to how intense you are in lifting the weights.

I remember my training partner, Jim Herman, back then. I had a couple of years of experience in weight training than him so therefore I was a little bit stronger. Both of us were making excellent progress not because of the amount of weights we were using, but because of our intensity. I recall the time when he and I were doing dumbbell presses for our chest. I was using a pair of 120lbs, while Jim was using a pair of 75lbs. I remember pressing those dumbbells till I couldn't anymore and I did 13 reps with it. Jim lifted his and did the same 13 reps. The intensity of our training was indeed the same since both of us couldn't do anymore than 13 reps. Sure I lifted more weights than him, but that's only because of my years of experience. He eventually caught up to me in weight usage. His motivation was indeed a big factor in this.

So it really doesn't matter if you are lifting 10lbs or 100lbs as long as the intensity is there. This part of the book probably left you with a lot of questions when it comes to training intensity, the duration of it, and its frequency. I promise things will become clearer as you read along.

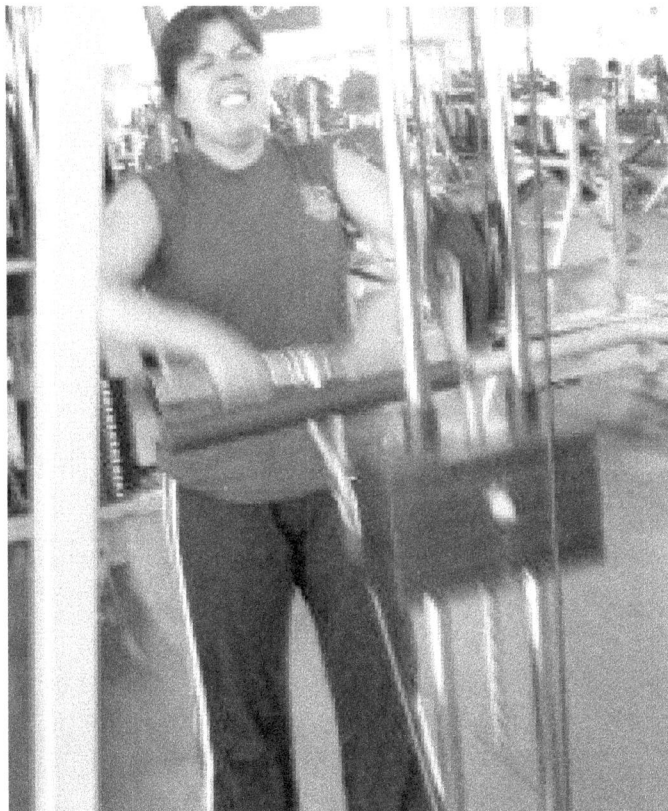

Adriana Garcia

Intensity is more important than how much you can lift.

CHAPTER 5

RECUPERATION

(Second Part in the Trinity)

I remember going in the locker room and seeing two of my gym buddies who I've known for a long time. They were discussing their workouts. One of them said to the other as he was laying out his plan for his back workout that day: "I'm gonna hit the T rows first and do 5 set of that, then I'm gonna do wide pulldowns to the back and do 5 set of that, then I'm gonna grab a 60lb dumbbell and do rows-I might go all the way up to 100lbs-I'm gonna have to see how I feel, you know what I mean? And then, I'm gonna finish my back by doing 3 sets of pull ups for 10 reps."

He turned to look at the mirror and flexed his back by doing a lat spread. "Yeah! Look at these babies! They are growing!"

"Hey man, how long are you gonna workout?" asked his buddy who's been listening to him attentively.

"I don't know, maybe 1 ½ to 2 hours at most. I have to do some biceps afterward and then I have to hit the treadmill for like 30 minutes," he answered as his enthusiasm died down when he started thinking about length of time he had to spend in the gym. "I guess I better get started. The old lady wouldn't want me coming home late."

They then turned their attention to me as they saw me finish putting on my workout attire. I was looking over at my training log that day. I wanted to see the exercises I was doing and how much weight I would be using.

"Hey Edgar, whatcha got going today, man?" The one who was talking about his workout asked me.

"I got legs today," I said to them.

"Oh yeah, what are you doing?"

"I'm doing a set of leg press, a set of leg extension, and a set of leg curls along with a set of calf raises."

"Wait a minute. Did you say A SET of leg press, A SET of leg extension, and A SET of leg curls?" asked his buddy.

"Yup, I'll be out of here in 15 minutes."

"What?" they both said with a look of disbelief on their faces.

"Is that how you grow?" his buddy asked me.

"That's how I grow."

The man who talked about his workout routine had a confuse look on his face. He then asked me, "Hey man, when are you actually gonna start working out?"

When I first joined the gym I had dreams and aspirations of becoming a competitive bodybuilder, just like the bodybuilders I've admired in the muscle magazines and books. I have trained 2 to 3 hours a day because the muscle magazines said that this was how champions trained. I also ate pretty much the same food and took the same supplements as they did.

I did made some progress, but for the amount of time I was putting in my workouts, the food I was eating, and the supplements I was taking my progress was mediocre at best. I was expecting more. I was expecting to add 2" to my arms, 4" to my chest, and 3" to my thighs just like the bodybuilders in the magazines claimed they've made on average with that type of training, eating and with those type of supplements. I thought if I followed them with a fine tooth comb I would make the same progress. Of course I later realized that all these bodybuilders who made these claims were taking huge quantity of anabolic drugs. The muscle magazines failed to mention that.

I've come to accept that I was mediocre. I was doomed to stay skinny for the rest of my life. Going to the gym and spending hours there, eating plain food, and wasting my money on supplements didn't appeal to me much anymore. It felt like I was giving away some part of my lifespan to working out. If it wasn't for Dr. Darden's book on *"The Nautilus Book"* I wouldn't have understood what proper training was all about and what it means to *recuperate* after training.

As I said before, your workout must be intense, short, and infrequent. There is a very good reason why your workout must be this way. It all has to do with recuperation. What exactly is recuperation you ask? Have you ever had a major cut, a sprained ankle, or fractured a bone? What do you do once you had it bandaged, wrapped, or put on a cast? You rest it. Rest or recuperation is the only way for it to get better. That's why when you do a H.I.T. workout it must be brief because your body can only tolerate so much of that intensity and it must be infrequent so that your body can be given a chance to recuperate before you engage in another H.I.T. workout.

High level of resistance training triggers recuperation to take place. Remember, your muscles have been stimulated by a H.I.T. workout, the moment you put down the weights recuperation immediately goes into action. This is why you don't grow in the gym as some trainers think. Growth takes place outside the gym, especially when you are at rest. It takes a certain amount of time to fully recuperate. If you were to go back to the gym again the next day to do the same H.I.T. workout then you would have disturbed your recuperation and therefore retarding your progress.

Recuperation is Systematic

When you go to the gym to workout your arms you should keep in mind that you are not only working out your arms, but pretty much your entire body. Even though the focal point of your workout is your arms; other muscles come into play such as your legs, shoulders, back, and such. Such muscles are called *stabilizer muscles.*

To some degree these stabilizer muscles are also getting a workout. When you are doing a H.I.T. they come into play even more. For example if you were doing barbell curls with 30lbs and it is too easy your legs, shoulders, back, and forearms are not so tense. Now if you were to jump into doing 100lb barbell curls then those stabilizer muscles would be more tense in order to make sure that your body stays steady while you perform that exercise.

Keep in mind as well the physiological aspect also comes into play. So going back to training arms again, when you are doing this you are using your whole body's energy supply. This is the reason why you may feel exhausted throughout your body after doing arms. There's so much to physiology and how it plays into this that for now we will only concern ourselves with energy and tissue (muscle) repair and how it plays into recuperation.

What was lost through your arms workout would have to be replenished plus more. This means that you recuperate locally at your arms and systematically from a physiological stand point. The plus more means that when your arm muscles fully recuperate 100% it is to hope that it has adapted to the stress of the exercise by getting stronger. So this means that you've given your system time to recuperate and the proper nutrients for it to take in so that full recovery and energy to the muscles are restored. This is why it's a big mistake to do another H.I.T. before recuperation is complete.

Overtraining and Undertraining

I remember having a conversation once with a health spa or gym sales rep. about the people who were signing up to join his gym. He was bragging to me how he signed up over 50 or so new members to his gym in one week at the beginning of the year (New Year's Resolution). I remember asking him, "Your gym must be packed?"

"Nah, I just give them 3 months and over 90% of them will be gone."

"Over 90% gone in 3 months, then your gym must be losing some money?"

"No, that's why we set up a one year contract with them, this way we continue to collect even when they are not going."

It's true that over 90% of the new members tend to drop out within the first 3 month. Many gyms tend to rely on this statistic in order to keep their profit margin going and to keep their gym going with new members all the time. Now imagine if all of the members who ever signed up decided to honor their 1 year contract by showing up all the time, there would be wall to wall people trying to workout, if they could even workout that is.

So why is that most new members tend to drop out within the first few months? The answer is quite simple, it's because they tend to overtrain. New members are usually enthusiastic, full of energy, and very motivated to workout in order to accomplish their fitness goal. The problem they have is how exactly do they approach their training.

I've seen new gym members before working out the same body parts every single day. I've seen some do 1 hour aerobics and 2 hours weight training. They have this mentality of training more is better. They soon quit because they burned out. Along with this burnt out feeling comes the loss of motivation and goal. Many realize that spending that much time in the gym and seeing very little result was not worth it.

This burned out feeling is what we define as overtraining. Once you have reached this state, progress comes to a halt and you may even regress. Your body feels drained all the time. Not only is your body drained, but so is your state of mind. Overtraining is not a very good feeling at all and if you continue to be in this state for a long time you may run yourself into some health risk. Such as prolonged tissue tear, dehydration, constant fatigue, dried skin, premature aging, high blood pressure, or immune problems which leads to constant illness.

When I used to have my own personal training business my problem was that every time I get a new client to train I had to keep their motivation in check. So you, as a person who is trying to get rid of your skinny self must do whatever you can to avoid overtraining. Keep in mind that overtraining kills progress. Your sure bet is to always undertrain.

Undertraining means to never exhaust your ability to fully recuperate. That means you go in the gym and do a H.I.T. workout just so you can trigger your muscles growth process in strength and size and then go home in order to allow recuperation to fully take place. It is to hope that once recuperation is complete that you would have added some strength and muscle mass to your body. Again: brief, intense, and infrequent is the key.

Lessen Your Physical Activities

I once had a client who stood 6'3" and weighed 160lbs. Now a person who is this tall and weighs this much is considered very thin. I've been seeing this man train in my gym for almost 10 years. And for those 10 years I have never seen him make any significant progress. He, on the other hand has seen me and the clients I've trained made progress over the years and he often complimented me for it.

One day he signed up for a couple of training session with me. He passionately told me how frustrated he was for his lack of progress and for being too thin. He said for almost 10 years he's been training he had only seen a gain of 5lbs. So that means he had gone from 155lbs to 160lbs. That is indeed discouraging and frustrating to invest all that time and energy only to see that much progress.

So I sat down with him and tried to schedule him. Scheduling him turned out to be the hardest thing. Along with his 40-50 hour a week job he plays minor league baseball. He goes to practice almost every evening after work. On top of that he goes out with his girlfriend to do mountain biking once or twice a week and even plays racquet ball with her. He also sometimes goes golfing with his friends in the weekend where he does a lot of walking he said. I asked him as to when he actually gets to do weight training and he said whenever he can.

This man's life very much centered around his physical activities. I flat out told him that his physical activities were killing his progress. He wasn't allowing his body to recuperate properly and therefore he was putting himself in a constant state of overtraining. I told him to ease up on it and to focus on weight training in order to achieve his physical goal of gaining muscle mass. He agreed and allowed me to train him for 3 months.

After 3 months he was quite pleased with the result. He asked me to train him for another 3 months. After 6 months of H.I.T. his weight went from 160lbs to 195lbs. He was satisfied being at this weight and so my training sessions with him ended. He often bragged to the guys in the gym that it was me who helped him gain mass and strength, but in actuality his easing up on those physical activities allowed his body to recuperate better and because of this his gains were very good.

If your goal is to get rid of your skinny self then you must prioritize weight training. I'm not saying that you should cut all your physical activities, but rather ease up on them. If your physical activities are just as strenuous as your weight training then you are using up your recuperative capability and putting yourself in a state of overtraining.

I, myself, enjoy cycling, hiking, and playing basketball, but these physical activities are more of a supplement to my weight training. I will never go all out on my cycling or go try a marathon. Only in weight training will I go all out.

Yes, in the past I have trained football players, swimmers, and other athletes before. Their goal is to become better at their sport. So in this case, weight training to them becomes supplemental. Yours should be the opposite. But if you want to be a football player or some other athlete in the near future and you want to get rid of your skinny self first, then focus on weight training for now till you reach your physical goal.

Sleep, the Ultimate Recuperation

If you are a working adult living in the United States then chances are you are one of the many Americans who doesn't get enough sleep. Because of a busy lifestyle many people only sleep 5 to 6 hours a day. Ideally the average person should be getting around 8 to 9 hours of sleep a day. It is said that people who get very little sleep tend to be less productive, irritable, and more vulnerable to illness. They basically have less energy during the day.

Doctors often put their seriously injured patients in a state of comatose for days in order to allow their body's own natural healing process to fully take place. Sleep is sort of the same way as well. The functions of your body slow down and allow recuperation to take place more efficiently. Cells throughout your body get rejuvenated, especially your muscle cells.

You must allow your body to enter into that deep sleep, in a state of *Rapid Eye Movement* (REM) in order to have full rest. You must invest at least 8 to 9 hours length of sleep in order to achieve proper recuperation. So in other words your sleep should be a recuperative sleep. Your dreams must be so deep that you somehow don't even know that you are in that dream state. In other words, your dreams should feel real.

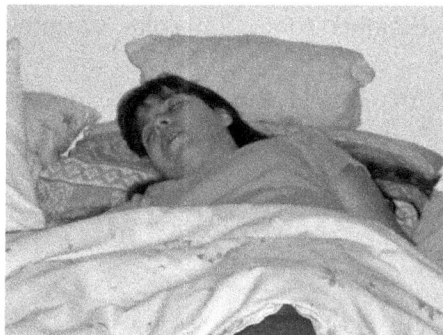

Adriana Garcia

Snoring, Insomnia, and taking Naps

Loud persistent snoring can be a problem. I recommend you see your doctor about this. This could mean that there might be some kind of health problem or even a health risk. Snoring doesn't mean that you are getting a full rest. Upon waking up you might often times still feel tired and sometimes with a headache.

It is said that 20-40% of the people in the United States suffer from insomnia. I've fallen into this category before myself. Often times it has something to do with too much stress and anxiety. If this is your problem then I suggest you see a doctor about it. He or she may prescribe proper sleeping aides for you.

Like I said, many working people in the U.S. don't get enough sleep at night. If this is true for you then I suggest you take naps during the day. I often refer to this as *power naps.* I tend to do this after work. I go straight to bed and take a 40 minute to an hour power nap. I even do this during my lunch break at work. I go to my car and recline the seat and just close my eyes and let my body relax completely while listening to classical music. I don't fall always fall asleep, but my mind do enter into a meditative state where I start to think I'm somewhere else, while my whole body feels very heavy and relax. It works! I feel great and more productive at work.

I never go straight to the gym after work, because my mind and my body would be too tired. Instead I take a nap first. I tend to have more energy and more focus for my workout after a nap. So if you're not getting sufficient night sleep, then take your power naps during the day.

CHAPTER 6

NUTRITION

(Third Part in the Trinity)

Nutrition is such a huge topic that this could have been a book in itself. There's just so much to discuss and to cover. I was rather hesitant if I should go ahead and add this topic to this book or to do it in a book by itself. I went ahead and decided to add it and talk about it briefly, because in way I didn't want to break up the *Trinity in Bodybuilding*. And this is the last part of that trinity. Just to let you know I will have this topic broken down into chapters so it would be easier to follow.

So you already know that high level of resistance training stimulates muscles to get stronger and to increase in size. You've come to know that once the muscles are stimulated you must allow recuperation to take place by not doing any high level resistance training or physical activities till this process is complete. Now you must come to know how important it is for nutritional supplies to be present in your body when your muscles demand for it during the exercise and during recuperation.

One good thing about living in the United States is that we don't have to worry about the lack of nutrition in our diet. There's an overabundance of nutrition in our diet. Unlike other countries that worry about not getting enough of it, we on the other hand have to worry about getting too much of it.

The average American does get more than enough *carbohydrate*, *protein*, and *fat* in their diet. There's hardly a case for malnutrition here unless they are purposefully doing it to themselves. If you still have doubts in your mind about not getting all the nutrients, especially if your diet consist of mostly meat and junk food then I would recommend you take a multi-vitamin and multi-mineral supplement once a day.

Scientists have categorized nutrients into two parts, *macro-nutrients* and *micro-nutrients*. Macro-nutrients refer to nutrients in food that has an energy value in a form of calories. These are the calories that come from carbohydrate, protein, and fat. Depending on the type of food you are eating and how much of it the amount of calories will vary. So if you are eating a chicken breast, over 90% of the calories you get from that would be from protein and the rest from fat. If you are eating rice then over 90% of the calories would be from carbohydrate and the rest from protein (incomplete protein). Now if you are drinking whole milk you can bet that more than half of the calories from it are from fat and the rest from protein and carbohydrates.

Micro-nutrients are vitamins and minerals. They do not have any energy value, but they are vital to the proper function of your body and to your well being. Unfortunately there's just too many of them to cover and this is the part that I will leave out in this book in order to make it brief. I highly recommend that you go to your local library or bookstore and checkout the books that are out there. Learn how important water soluble and fat soluble vitamins are and what different type of minerals do for you. Learn too what electrolytes such as *potassium* and *sodium* does for you.

Since micro-nutrients are not covered I would like to instill in your mind though to always eat foods that are dense in vitamins and minerals such as fresh fruits, vegetables, whole wheat, legumes, and grains. Stay away or only eat occasional process foods that are caloric dense and have less micro-nutrient value such as various junk foods. The diet plan in this book will ensure that you are getting all the proper nutrients that your body needs.

Macro-Nutrients

I remember being in 5th grade in the mid-80's and how we were required to take the physical fitness test where we run, do sit ups, pull ups, push ups, and such. I remember my teacher Mrs. Ursino saying to her colleague how the fitness level of the children seemed to be getting worse and worse as time passes. She was right. Today the United States has an obesity crisis especially among our children and the culprit seems to be carbs (short for carbohydrate) enriched foods. Back in the 80's it was fat enriched foods that was blamed, but today it's carbs. In truth, neither carbs nor fat are to blame. It's the huge servings that have quadrupled over the past few decades are to blame along with the lack of physical activities due to the conveniences technology has brought to us. Of course you don't have to worry about this crisis because you are trying to get rid of your skinny self through bodybuilding, but its good information to have anyway, in case you care.

CHAPTER 7

CARBOHYDRATE

This macro-nutrient is your body's prime source of energy, especially to the brain and hard working muscles. Basically carbohydrates that enter into your body are broken down into tiny molecules. Each of these molecules goes into your body's Krebs Cycle and gets converted into an energy source for your muscles in a form of ATP. Without getting into too much detail, just keep in mind that carbohydrate is your main fuel for your workout. It's also what your brain prefers when it comes to nourishment. So if you want power and strength during your workout and some intelligence eat carbs.

There are 3 basic forms to carbohydrate: complex, simple, and fiber. Your diet should consist of mostly complex carbs. This is sort of like the battery that last for a very long time in your body. Endurance athletes such as marathon runners, cyclist, swimmers, and so forth rely on this macro-nutrient for their energy. Bodybuilders such as yourself rely on this to power your workouts and also to help keep your digestive system healthy and regular. If you hear a gym rat talk about how protein powers up his workout then I suggest you smile courteously and walk away. You know better that it is carbs that does that.

Complex Carbohydrate

It is often referred to as *starch* or *polysaccharides* consisting of long chains of sugar molecules that are linked together. Good sources are found in foods such as rice, whole grain, wheat, beans, oats, potatoes, and certain vegetables. Once in the body carbs are converted into a molecule known as *glycogen* and they are often times stored in the muscles and in the liver. This particular molecule needs water as its medium. One molecule of carb would need 4 molecules of water. This is good, because as you know muscles are well over 70% water. This is going to make your muscles look fuller. People who go on high protein, low carbs, and low fat diet often times their muscles look flat and small. I'm willing to bet that their workouts are not as strong and energetic as it should be.

Simple Carbohydrate

This is the opposite of complex carbohydrate when it comes to being a battery that is long lasting. Simple carbs are actually very short when it comes to energy. I remember working 10 hours straight at work without taking a break. I was starving and my brain was fried. I remember I had a chocolate bar in my locker. I ate it and in a few minutes my energy level was back up again. But after an hour pass my energy level dropped significantly and it literally felt like I hit a wall. If you plan on eating simple carb foods such as a candy bar then I suggest that you eat complex carbs before or along with that. Yes, stay away from those glazed donuts that your co-workers often times bring to work in the morning, especially if you haven't had a healthy breakfast of complex carbs and even if you did stay away from it anyway.

Simple carbs are also referred to as monosaccharides (single unit sugar) and disaccharides (double unit sugar). They are found in foods such as fruits, candies, and just about anything that taste sweet. So does this mean fruits and candies and anything sweet are bad for you? That depends. Fruits as we know since elementary school are good for you. They are nutrient dense and the type of sugar that they have (mostly fructose) does not spike up the sugar level in your body and they are low in calories.

Candies and other sweets on the other hand are high calories made from sugar and they should be eaten in moderation. They lack any significant nutrients and they can spike up your sugar level. They often times don't get stored like complex carbs do, unless eaten in excess then they are converted into fat. As a bodybuilder this won't be beneficial to you, but it's alright to eat them in moderation.

Fiber

About thirty years ago there was a cereal commercial in TV where the actors were trying to figure out or remember the second word that was on the cereal box: "It's Fruit and...?" The word they were looking for was "fiber." I often laugh when I see this commercial, because a good amount of fiber will send you straight to the toilet. So how on earth could anyone forget the word "fiber" in the "Fruit and Fiber" cereal box is beyond me.

Fiber by itself is not an energy source. It does not elevate your sugar level nor does it breakdown into anything. It basically helps you with your elimination and maintaining homeostasis (balance) in your body. Fiber is found in mostly carb source foods. It is found in foods such as oatmeal, bake beans, applesauce, apple, celery, many cereals, and other natural, non-meat food products.

These are the many benefits of fiber:

- Protection from constipation by initiating bowel movement.

- Protection from colon and rectal cancer by preventing precancerous growth

- Protection from diverticulosis which is the development of tiny bulges that can cause painful constipation.

- Protection from heart disease by lowering the bad cholesterol in the body known as LDL (Low Density Lipids).

- Protection from obesity, because foods rich in fiber promotes satiates (feeling full or satisfied) where you will be less likely to eat more.

- Protection from diabetes which reduces the need for insulin because it slows down the absorption of carbs in your intestine.

Protein Sparing

This is another very good reason why you must never sacrifice your carb consumption in order to avoid using protein as your energy source. So, when you hear someone say that you should eat more protein than carbs in order to build muscle strength and mass, again just smile courteously and walk away. They really don't know what they're talking about. I don't recommend that you donate part of your lifespan listening to them lecture you on this.

Protein and carbs do give out the same energy value which is 4 calories per 1 gram. So yes, both of them are energy source. But unlike carb, protein is not only an energy source, but a builder of tissue, particularly muscle tissue. Its primary duty is to repair. So when you are recuperating, protein is playing a major role in that.

So for many people who have a diet consisting of less than 60 grams of carbs a day, especially to those who work out, they will make their bodies use protein as an energy source in order to make up for the missing carbs. A lack of sufficient carb is called *ketosis*. You don't want your body to use protein as its prime energy source because it would retard the muscle building strength and mass during recuperation. This is why your calorie intake should be 60% carbs and 30% protein and the rest fat. Your body prefers carb as its energy and protein for tissue repair. So never cut off your carb consumption in favor of eating more protein.

Oxidation of Fat

Since carb is your body's primary energy source it also helps to burn off the fat. Our body is far more efficient than any machinery out there when it comes to energy. Appliances rely on electricity for its energy source. Once the plug is pulled the appliance seizes to function. Same thing with our cars, once the fuel is out our cars won't run. There's no such thing as a reserve tank or reserve electricity, but we do. We have stored fat that burns along with our carbs.

Imagine yourself camping. You wanted to build a bonfire. You gathered a couple of logs. Now you can't just turn on your lighter or light a match and try to burn them. The logs are too big and too dense to be lit up. What you need are twigs. You place the twigs around and underneath the logs. You light up the twigs first. Once they are burning the logs will start to slowly burn as well and pretty soon they will be the only ones that are burning. Logs will burn for a long time while the twigs will soon burn off.

Fat serves you the same way when it comes to long lasting energy. Carbs serve as a

starter and soon the fat will burn along with it. This is why you are able to walk for miles

and miles without stopping to eat. This is why marathon runners can run up to 26 miles

and cyclist up to 300 hundred miles.

So how does this relate to resistance training? It doesn't. Your body will

primarily use carbs only during your hard workout. But once you finish your workout

and you return to your daily activities it does make your body more efficient in burning

or using fat, even when you're asleep. This means that you have improved your

metabolism (a process in which we use food to create energy to sustain the functions of

our body).

CHAPTER 8

PROTEIN

Unlike fat and carbohydrate that has gotten a bum rap over the past few decades, protein has received nothing but praises. Fitness industries and so-called nutrition experts have pushed the notion in our heads that we need to eat more protein. Are they right?

If you live in the United States then chances are you are not protein deprived. The average American eats 3 to 5 times the amount of protein requirement a day. Compare to other nations like Europe, we are eating 2 times more protein than they do on average a day and compare to impoverished nations such as third world countries we are eating 8 to 12 times more than them.

My American friend who was originally from India and is a diehard *vegan* is not protein deprived. He learned to mix his nuts, grains, legume, vegetables, and tofu in a certain way in order to get all the necessary protein he needs a day. The only way a person in the U.S. can be lacking protein in their diet would be if they did it on purpose. So throw away this notion that you might be protein deprived.

If you are working out then your protein needs would be more than that of the average sedentary person. How much more is very hard to tell. It all depends on our metabolism and how much our muscles need it during recuperation. So what is the best way of knowing? I once heard of using a nitrogen strip to measure the acidity in our urine in order to find out how much protein we need. This is not entirely true, because if your urine is too acidic then that means you are using protein for energy instead of carbs.

I've heard of other ways too like blood test, a straight urine test after a hard workout, BMR (basal metabolic rest) test and so on. Unfortunately, these so-called tests can be inaccurate.

What the RDA Recommends and What I Recommend

Basically to figure out the amount of protein you need a day the RDA recommends that you take your weight by pounds and divide that by 2.2. This will put your weight in kilograms (a standard of measure that most countries use). Then you multiply that by 0.8. The answer from this would be your required daily intake.

So let's say that you weigh 150lbs.

150 divided by 2.2 = 68kg.   Now 68 multiply by 0.8 = 54

So according to the RDA you should eat about 54 grams of protein a day. That is if you are a sedentary person. Now an 8oz chicken breast has more protein than that.

Now the RDA will probably lynch me for saying this, but for a person who is a bodybuilder that is just too low. You would need twice that amount to build up your muscles. So if you are 150lbs I would recommend that you multiply that 54 by 2. So that means you should be eating 108g of protein a day. But like I said, if you're an American, you are probably getting far more than 108g of protein a day. Believe it or not even what I'm recommending to you would still be considered too low by those muscle magazines standards.

But if you are in doubt just be sure that you are getting 20-30 grams of protein per meal. If you are eating 5 times a day and if you are getting this amount then you are in good shape. Just be sure that the proteins are from a good source such as meat, poultry, fish, and dairy.

Amino Acid

These are the building blocks for protein, just as polysaccharides are for carbs. Amino acids are linked together like beads or chains. All and all there are about 22 different kinds of amino acids. It's not necessary to know each of them and their functions, but know that 8 out of those 22 amino acids we can not manufacture in our bodies. So those 8 are known as *essential amino acids*. We have to make sure that we obtain them from our diet. If you're eating those protein sources that I mentioned in this book then you don't have to worry.

Complete and Incomplete

Complete protein usually refers to having all the 22 amino acids present, especially the essential amino acids. Again, complete proteins are found in fish, poultry, meat, and dairy. Incomplete protein refers to proteins that are missing 1, 2, 3 or more of the essential amino acids. *Incomplete proteins* are usually found mostly in vegetable sources.

Now if you're a vegetarian don't worry. You can combine different kinds of vegetables together in order to make it into a complete protein. By combining baked beans with rice, peanut butter with wheat bread, soy with corn, and so forth. These types of combination are referred to as *complimentary protein*. The only problem with complimentary protein is that you have to eat more of it in order to get the same dosage as that of a person who eats meat.

Protein and Amino Acid Supplements

I get a lot of questions on taking protein and amino acid supplements when I used to be a personal trainer and when I used to compete in natural bodybuilding shows and even on my websites. I never recommended taking just protein supplements by themselves, because our body usually prefers a complete meal over just protein. We assimilate the nutrients better and we have more energy. Protein by itself just doesn't do that. If you do plan on taking Protein supplement in a powder form then I recommend you add a banana to it to make it as a meal.

Once you consume the protein it goes to the stomach for digestion and then gets broken down in our intestines by these enzymes known as peptidases. These enzymes break the protein into individual amino acids which passes through the intestinal wall and make its way into our bloodstream. Most of it is stored in the liver and or if they are in excess they are converted as fat.

Protein as a meal along with carbs and some fat works better for our body. This is because our body functions in a synergistic way. There are different enzymes present in our body and because of the need of our body it is better to have all macro-nutrients present, instead of just one. In other words our body is never hungry for just protein alone. It wants the whole thing. If you need a snack for a meal then snack on some of the high protein bars or Protein shakes that are out there with you adding a banana to it. Many of them have 15-20 grams of complete protein, which is good.

Amino acid Supplements are a waste of money. I remember during my teenage years part of my pay that I got from working at a fast food restaurant went into buying amino acid supplements. Come to find out later that they are not only a waste of money, but not really necessary. If you are eating a protein meal, then rest assure that you are getting all the amino acids you need.

Muscle magazines nowadays try to push for this amino acid supplements. They advertise it with champion bodybuilders who confessed that amino acid supplements worked great for them. Majority of these bodybuilders are on steroids anyway and any of the advertising they do serves as an income for them. Chances are they might not have ever used the product before or not at all.

My nutrition teacher once told me, "If you want amino acid supplements to work best, then you're going to have to inject it into your bloodstream." It makes sense because protein enters our mouth, gets digested in our stomach, and gets broken down into amino acid in our intestines by enzymes before it even goes into our bloodstream.

Mega-dosing on Protein

I got an email from a lady from Poland once. She told me that she was once a competitive bodybuilder and would like to go back to that sport again. When she sent me current pictures of herself the first thing that came out of my mouth was, "Wow, she's very thick!" She wasn't fat like a normal person would be; her fat was more evenly distributed throughout her body. In other words, she was very thick like a power-lifter.

She does diet and eats well. But the problem was that she was eating over 400 grams of protein day! I kid you not! Her diet was based on mostly protein which was by way of eating meat and eggs along with a number of protein powder supplements. Now for a lady that's 5'1" and weighs 175lbs that is way too much protein. Not to mention she was having all sorts of digestive and elimination problems.

I responded back by recommending she cut her protein intake significantly and increase her calories on complex carbs to make up for the missing calories from the protein. Sure enough she did lose some weight and was able to bring her bodyweight down to 125lbs and her body's definition was coming out. The problem was that she associated her weight loss to muscle loss because of the fewer amount of protein she was eating, which was around 100 grams a day. She ended up quitting my program. She was only 10 lbs away from her competitive form.

Most bodybuilders, especially those who are beginners, think that if you eat more protein the more muscles you'll developed. That is far from the truth. Your body will only take what it needs and the rest are stored in the liver. The liver in turn will convert this into fat, which gets stored throughout our body, such was the case for this lady from Poland.

CHAPTER 9

FAT

Fat, sometimes referred to as lipids, is an essential part of our diet. It carries the essential vitamins that our body needs such as A, D, E, and K. Fat gives us a feeling of satiety after eating. It is slow to digest and it holds back the feeling of hunger vs. a fat free or a low fat diet that leaves you feeling hungry after a couple of hours of eating. One good thing about fat is that you don't have to worry about not getting enough of it, you only have to worry about getting too much of it.

Fat as you know has had a bum rap over the past decades. For years people associated fat consumption with obesity, type II diabetes, cholesterol, strokes, heart disease, and so on. The health industry has made a lot of profit promoting fat free snacks, low fat diet meals, and so called diet pills that's suppose to suppress fat from being digested. Many of these are not accurate and some are down right false.

Though it is true that most of us do need to reduce fat from our diet in order to stay healthy, it isn't wise though to totally eliminate them. If you totally eliminate fat from your diet you will be missing out on those essential vitamins and some of the health benefits that fat can give you.

Fat does have over twice the caloric value compare to carbs and protein. One gram of fat is equal to 9 calories, vs. the 4 calories that you get from one gram of carbs and protein. So it is understandable why eating too much fat can make you obese. It is because of the calories which your body doesn't need gets stored as fat. But if you eat fat in a controlled way then you are fine.

Saturated and Unsaturated

You've probably heard of saturated and unsaturated. It's been used a lot by fitness gurus, but you're probably not quite certain as to what exactly they are. First, let's look at the fat molecule. A fat molecule consists of *glycerine* and 3 *fatty acids*. The 3 fatty acids are linked to the glycerine. How carbon and hydrogen atom attaches itself to fat chains will determine whether if it is saturated or unsaturated.

The most important thing you need to know is that saturated fat comes generally from animal source as well as dairy products. It is usually solid in room temperature. This is the type of fat many fitness gurus will tell you to stay away from and rightly so. Although they do add flavor to your meat, you must be careful not to eat too much of this. Because it carries with it some bad cholesterol that can lead to plaque build up in your arteries, which can cause serious health problems such as strokes or heart attack.

Unsaturated fat holds more hydrogen atoms than saturated and they generally come from plant source such as vegetables, safflower, peanuts, olives, soybeans, coconut, avocado, and so forth. They are usually liquid in room temperature. The liquid form is what we often use in cooking. For the most part unsaturated fat doesn't seem to raise the bad cholesterol that can cause plaque build up in our arteries.

Monounsaturated and Polyunsaturated

The day of cooking our food with lard (animal fat, mostly from pigs) is a thing of a past now. Growing up as a little boy in the Philippines, I remember my mom using this as her means to fry meat, especially chicken. I remember how tasty the foods were.

Then suddenly she switched to frying with canola oil because she heard that cooking with lard can cause heart attack and stroke. I remember missing that tasty fried chicken.

Since you understand now that unsaturated fat compared to saturated fat is better for you, especially when it comes to cooking, let me explain the 2 types of unsaturated. *Polyunsaturated* usually comes from corn, soybeans, cottonseed, and safflower. They are a couple of pair of hydrogen away from becoming saturated fat. *Monounsaturated* usually comes from olive, peanut, coconut, and avocado. *Monounsaturated* is only a pair of hydrogen away of becoming saturated fat. For decades it was debated as to which one is better for us, because one has a tendency of lowering the bad cholesterol (LDL) while increasing the good one (HDL) and the other has the tendency of increasing the bad one while decreasing the good one.

I remember in the 1980's that scientist and fitness gurus pushed for people to buy and use polyunsaturated oil, because it was believed to be better than monounsaturated oil. I remember it being pricey than the other oil. Then in the 1990's there was a big switch. All of a sudden scientist and fitness gurus were pushing for people to buy and use monounsaturated oil. And guess what, now it is that one that became pricey than the other. Yup, the principle of supply and demand.

Why is that? Because research has gotten better and it has now been concluded that monounsaturated actually promotes good cholesterol, while decreasing bad ones. Even though this seems to be the conclusion, stores are still selling and promoting polyunsaturated oil. They have become the poor man's choice for cooking. But still, people do buy them because in my opinion they taste better in cooking food with than monounsaturated oil.

HDL and LDL

So what exactly is good cholesterol and bad cholesterol?

Let's go back and look at fat again. Fat circulating in our body is known as *triglyceride*. When we eat too many calories that our body don't need they usually go to the liver and from there they can get converted into triglyceride. The triglyceride can then circulate in our body and gets stored in places where we don't want them. Usually the storage area in our body is determined by our genes. If your family has the tendency of storing fat in the belly or hips then chances are that's where yours will go first.

Now about 6-8% of that body fat is not all triglyceride, it is cholesterol. This is where it gets bad. Cholesterol often times accumulates in the inner wall of our arteries, causing plaque to build up. Bad cholesterol circulating in our body can be metabolized and eliminated by our liver. How? by a *lipoprotein* transport facilitator known as HDL (High Density Lipoprotein). Now cholesterol that doesn't get eliminated but rather transported into our body's cells, which can lead to accumulation in the arteries, is called LDL (Low Density Lipoprotein). It is very important that HDL be higher in ratio than LDL. The good news for you is that skinny people who do H.I.T. workouts and eats well tend to have high HDL level.

Dark Meat vs. White Meat

Fat is present in a lot foods we eat, especially in meat. Meat that tends to have a lot of the fat is called dark meat and meat that tends to be lean in fat is called white meat. Take for example chicken: legs and thighs are known as the dark part of the meat and breasts are known as the white part of the meat.

Dark meat tends to taste better than white meat. Like I mentioned before, fat has the tendency of making the meat taste good. White meat tends to be dry and sometimes dull to eat, but they are better for you than dark meat.

If you're like me and you much rather eat the dark meat then there is something you can do, trim off the fat. For example, take the skin off the chicken and cut off the excess fat around it. That will reduce the fat substantially. It still won't be as lean as white meat, but at least you'll get to enjoy your meal without eating too much fat.

Fat in Your Body

When I used to compete the lowest percentage of body fat I have ever had was 2.3%-3.6%. This was according to the caliper that was used on me by someone who has done this for decades. Of course, this might not be accurate, but for me it was consistent since I used the same person who measured me for both off and on seasons. Normally back then I would around 8% to 11% in my off seasons, but in my on seasons I could get very low.

I remember when I was preparing to compete in Natural USA bodybuilding contest and I wanted to come in lean and ripped. I remember my skin being paper thin. It didn't feel good to be very low in body fat. I was constantly cold even though the weather might be 80 degrees. I remember how easily I bruised and how easily I got tired. My workouts were weak too. For some of you who are painfully thin you probably know what I'm talking about. A comfortable percentage of body fat for me was indeed around 8% and above.

These are some of the most important things that fat in our body can do for us:

- Stored Energy – fat is our primary energy source when we are at rest. When we are doing moderate aerobics 70-80% of the energy used comes from fat. If our body is not getting enough calories to sustain itself then it will take it from our stored fat.

- Vitamins – fat is important when it comes to absorption of vitamin A, D, E, and K.

- Insulation – fat will help to keep us warm by preventing excess heat from escaping our body when the environment is cold.

- Protection – fat will help cushion any blows that might hit us. Fat also forms around our vital organs in order to prevent them from being injured.

CHAPTER 10

UNDERSTANDING CALORIE INTAKE

Now that you know that calories come from 3 different sources: carbs, protein, and fat, the next step is to know how much of it you need a day. Calories are energy value that are either used or stored. Remember, it takes energy to workout, energy to recuperate, energy to grow strong and to develop, and energy to sustain it.

In the U.S. I have talked about how people have been becoming obese due to calorie rich foods that come from large servings. Compare to other nations, America is indeed leading the way in obesity. This epidemic has reached our children for the past few decades. Their fitness level has gone down as well due to the lack of physical activities. Because of this we are now seeing all sorts of health problems from people who are eating too many calories. Doctors often times call this *metabolic disease*. But what about people like you? Where no matter how many calories you eat you can't seem to gain weight. There are perhaps some of you who are not eating properly and others who are not eating enough at all. Below are some of the reasons why you are thin:

Fast Metabolism

I recall a young man once asking this famous bodybuilder about his problem gaining weight because of his fast metabolism. The famous bodybuilder simply answered him, "Consider yourself blessed." That was all he ever said to him. It was not the answer that the young man was looking for, because he left the building feeling disappointed. I'm pretty sure this young man didn't vote for this famous bodybuilder to become the next governor of California.

Though one thing is true, it is better to have a fast metabolism than a slow one. You immediately burn up whatever food you eat. You are least likely to develop any health problems. But you are indeed stuck with a very skinny body. No matter how much exercise you do you still wound up skinny. In fact you may even wound up becoming skinnier than before, because exercise tends to burn up calories.

Here's what you must do. Log everything you eat, including the water you drink for at least 3 days. Then get a *food index book* and get a rough estimation as to how many calories you are eating a day. Rough estimation means that it is not exactly accurate, but it will give you some idea as to how many calories it takes to sustain you. Now from those 3 days you've counted your calories get the average rough estimation from that.

For example:

Day 1   Day 2   Day 3

2234 cal.   2878 cal.   2543 cal.

Now add them up:

2234 + 2878 + 2543 = 7655

Now divide 7655 by 3 and that comes out to 2552.

So this means that your average calories a day is roughly around 2552. This is how many calories it takes to sustain you and your daily activities, including your workouts.

My recommendation to you would be to add another 500 calories to your meals. So this means that you need to eat an average of 3052 calories a day. This can be achieved by either adding another meal or by increasing your servings. This *positive calorie* would be useful for your strength and mass gain. It will certainly give you more energy to do your workouts. Roughly about 60% of your total calories a day should be from mostly complex carbs, 30% from protein, and 10% from fat.

Poor Eating Habits

This was my problem back then when I used to weigh 118lbs and it might be yours as well, I had very poor eating habits. Usually poor eating habits can lead to obesity, but in cases like mine and perhaps yours it led us to being poorly developed. Back then I tend to eat junk foods that were empty in calories (lacking of any essential vitamins and minerals) as my meals. Eating in such a way causes the muscles to not get all the nutrients they need to develop themselves. So like me you'll end up looking like a soft, thin, pale, underdeveloped, unhealthy person who is very vulnerable to all kinds of illness, which I was often sick when I was young.

If this is the main reason why you are painfully thin then you must change your eating habits. Believe it or not this is extremely difficult for a lot of people. Why, because poor eating habits are something a person easily gets accustom too over the years. But if done gradually this poor eating habit can be broken.

I would say, give yourself 2 months to break away from the poor eating habits. Start substituting healthy food for junk food. For example: whole wheat bread for white bread, rice and beans for mash potatoes and gravy, grilled meat for deep fried meat, fruits for chips, protein meal bar for chocolate candy bar, and so on.

Once you've made this transition you'll discover that you actually feel better about yourself and you'll have more energy and vitality. Your body, especially your muscles, will crave more for these healthy foods, instead of your taste bud craving for those unhealthy ones.

Not Eating Enough

I've known people in the gym and outside the gym who only eat once or twice a day. Some of them believe that this would be the best way in keeping the fat weight off, while others are just too busy to eat. I'm assuming that many of you who are painfully thin are this way because you are too busy to eat. There may be some of you who just don't like to eat at all; believe it or not this is true of some people.

In any case you do have to find a way to at least eat 4 to 5 times a day. This is achievable even on a busy schedule. You just have to get used to preparing your food and carrying it around with you in a lunch box. I remember going to college full-time, working full-time, going to the gym, and doing homeworks in-between. Where ever I go, my food came along with me. Whenever I took my breaks at work I would eat, on my way to school I would eat, before and after the gym I would eat, and during the time I was doing my homework I would eat.

70

Sure I did eat out once in awhile, mostly in fast food restaurants, but that got to be too expensive. Most of these fast food places are not too keen on your health. Plus, waiting for them to prepare it was costing me precious time. Sure preparing your food the night before can be a chore, but the health benefits you get from it and the gains you achieve from your bodybuilding workouts make it worth the while.

I know there are people who are busier still and they can't manage to get 4 or 5 meals a day. In that case you can still eat 2 or 3 meals a day. Just be sure that the calories are there and it is a balance diet. There really is no proof that eating 4 or 5 meals a day is better than 2 or 3 meals day. It's just that 2 or 3 meals a day would be quite large by comparison and you might end up feeling too full and bloated.

Now if you don't like eating then you're going to have to literally force feed yourself. I know that there are some people out there that don't like to eat because they've associated food to something negative. If this is true for you then I recommend you see your doctor. It may be psychological or it can even be a chemical imbalance in your brain.

CHAPTER 11

GAINING WEIGHT

I can easily tell you to eat everything on the table, except for the utensils and plate just so you can gain weight in whatever way possible, but that wouldn't be wise. You've already read that too many calories can lead to fat storage and can be a risk to your health. I know some of you welcome a little bit of fat development and that is alright. A little bit of fat on your body is not a bad thing. There are health benefits to it compare to being painfully thin.

Stay away from so-called weight gainer supplements. These supplements tend to be very high in carbs, especially in simple carbs. They have the tendency of spiking up your sugar and insulin level. You can get a crash and burn feeling from this. They also tend to be very high in protein. You now know that too much protein which the body doesn't use or need tend to be stored as fat. Most of all, weight gainer supplements are extremely high in calories.

Many weight gainer supplements tend to pride themselves on the amount of calories they can supply over the other brands. The last time I went to the health food store I saw a weight gainer supplement that can give you 5000 calories per 2 servings. That is just too extreme and you bet this will not lead you to having better gains. Only your fat cells will gain from this.

If you are looking for another meal and you want it to be drinkable then I recommend a balance shake meal. You can get this at the grocery stores, pharmacy counter, and health food stores. Read the label and make sure all the essential vitamins and minerals are there. Make sure that the carbs are from a complex source, be sure that the protein is somewhere between 20 and 30 grams and are complete, and the fat at a minimum.

The Best Way to Gain Weight

If you gained 15-20lbs of weight in your first year of bodybuilding training through H.I.T. and diet then your result is excellent. The 2nd year you may gain 10-15lbs and you hope for the 3rd year to be the same. As you become more and more advance the gains tend to slow down and that is completely natural. At the advance level if you gain 5-10lbs in a year that is considered a great progress. Your body can only develop so much that it tends to slow down in time, so do expect this to happen.

But it does take a long time to reach that level of development and a lot of people, including myself, have not yet reached that level. So don't worry if you think that there's nothing to look forward to once you're there. It takes years of training to reach your goal. I've known people in their 50's and they feel that they haven't yet reached their full development.

It is very important that you always assess your progress and make adjustments to your nutritional needs, particularly in the calorie part. Going back to the example of eating 3052 calories to sustain you, your workouts, and your gains, let's say that your progress has plateau and you were eating this many calories. You haven't gained any weight at all in awhile now. Then it's time to add another 300 calories a day to your meals. So this means your average consumption of calories would be at 3352. This will help you continue in gaining weight, hopefully by way of muscles. Do monitor and see if the added calories are going to your muscles and not to your fat storage. If it's going to

your fat then adjust the calories by lowering it to 3100-3150. We want the gains to be

muscles as much as possible.

Be patient with your gains! Just remember, Rome wasn't

built in day.

CHAPTER 12

EATING OUT

Eating out once in a while is alright, but making a habit of eating out every single day is bad for you. Why, because eating out is truly a gamble. No matter which restaurants you go too, you really don't know what they've put in their foods. Even those so-called salad places, which we tend to think is safe, we often times don't know how well they've washed those vegetables or how much sodium are in their salad dressings.

Restaurants tend to use a lot of salt and fat in their food in order to make them tasty and to give you that full satisfied feeling. Even in salads they use dressings that are high in salt and calories. The servings are usually big in order to attract you and to have you feeling full. You truly have no control over how they prepare their food, but if you must eat out for the sake of getting your calories in then there are ways.

You can certainly select the healthiest meal from their menu. Usually, these are the meals that have vegetables, salads, grilled or baked meat, and grains. Instead of ordering a hamburger, order a chicken sandwich. Instead of eating fries, eat fruit salad. Instead of eating ice cream, eat yogurt. Instead of drinking a soda, drink water.

If you are to eat in a restaurant that gives huge servings, then be sure to have a to-go-box next to you. Just because it's on your plate doesn't mean you have to finish the whole thing. Often times huge servings tend to have over 2,000 calories in them that you're not aware of. That's enough calories to feed 3 supermodels for a whole day.

It's alright to give yourself a break and splurge on whatever food you want. This is usually called *cheat day*. You can do this once or twice a week. On the day you decide to do this be sure to adjust your meals by subtracting from it. For example, if I decided to eat at an Italian restaurant today for dinner then I will go ahead and skip a meal or two earlier in the day. For example I may skip my protein meal and my afternoon snack. I may even eat a light lunch. This way you don't introduce too many calories to your body in one day. Because too many calories from a meal that is somewhat unhealthy can make you feel sluggish throughout the day that can even go onto the next day. And you can definitely feel it in your workouts.

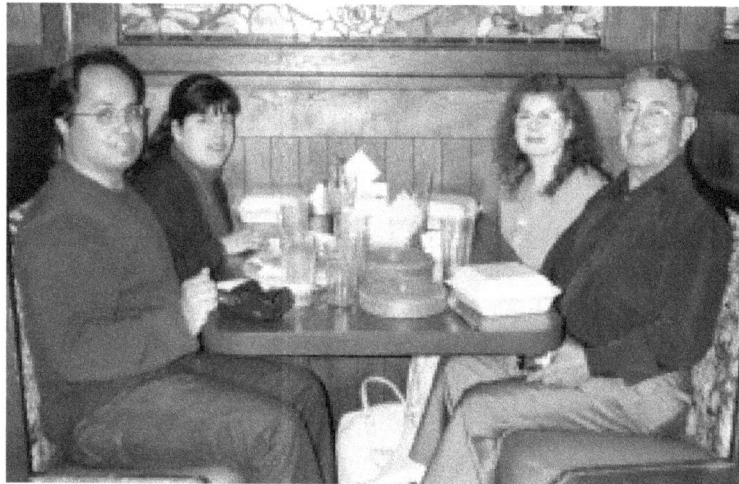

At a restaurant with our to-go-boxes.

CHAPTER 13

ETHNIC FOODS

Most foods that people eat are very much in line with their culture. I'm Filipino by decent and I was fortunate to have a good mom who cooked good food. When I was living at home I was eating rice, chicken, fish, and vegetables, all prepared and cooked according to my culture. Most ethnic foods are healthy, but you do need to watch out for some of the bad ones.

In my culture, pig is considered a luxury food, while fish and chicken are for the poor. But health wise we know that eating too much pig and eating the wrong parts from it is bad for your health. Another thing you have to watch out for are the spices that are used to prepare the food. They can have too much sodium that can lead to hypertension in the long run. So if you do eat according to your culture then make sure you prepare your food in the healthiest way possible. Learn to use salt substitute such as herbs and spices and use high sodium spices sparingly and watch the fat.

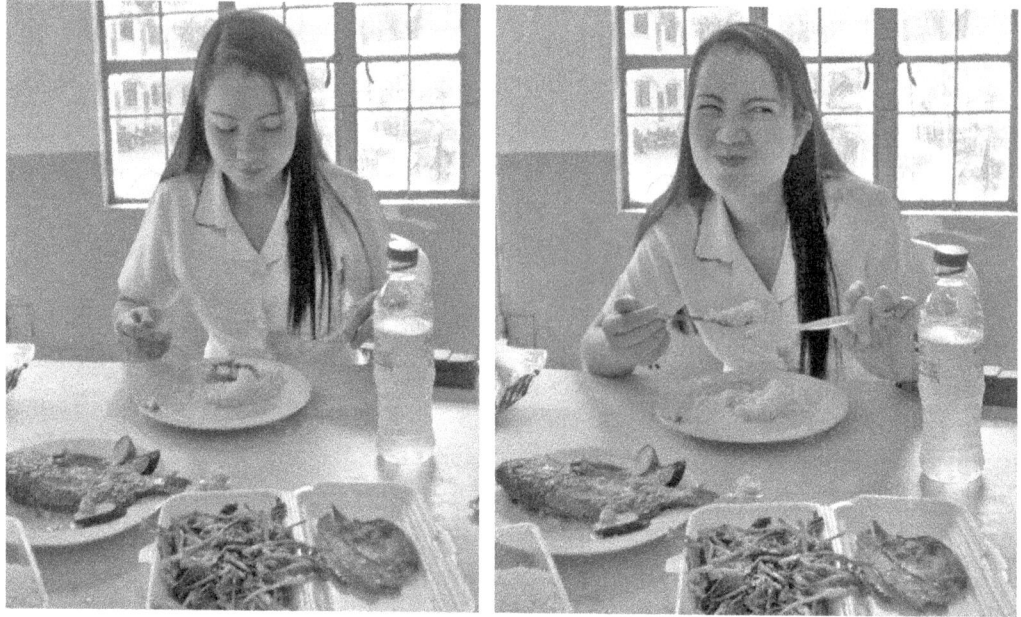

In many ways cultural foods are healthy, which is what my Filipina wife, Shiela Garcia, is eating.

CHAPTER 14

SUPPLEMENTS

In the past I have often been asked about this as to what supplements I take. I always surprise people when I tell them that I only take a multi-vitamin and mineral, protein meal, and occasionally creatine. For some reason they think that I should be taking in more supplements in order to be a complete bodybuilder. I tell them that hard training, followed by recuperation and proper nutrition is all that is needed to be a complete bodybuilder. Most of them don't seem to accept this Trinitarian Principle.

I can understand why most trainers have the mentality that they need supplements in order to achieve their goal, because the muscle magazines told them so. If you look at any muscle magazines lately you'll see that 30% of their content is based on advertising bodybuilding supplements. This is how the fitness industries make their profit. They like to show before and after photos of professional bodybuilders and fitness individuals as their models to sell their products. These models swear that it works. Most of these models might have taken these supplements, but they also took steroids and other drugs on top of that. Some of these models purposefully allowed themselves to get out of shape so they could take the before pictures and then hit the weights and the drugs hard in order to take the after pictures. Some might even do it in reverse where they take pictures of them when they are in top shape as an *after picture* and then allow themselves to get out of shapes so pictures could be taken of them and use it as their *before picture*. Yes, sad but true, most of these model bodybuilders and fitness individuals make their living off of being spoke persons for these supplement companies.

When I was fresh out of high school I landed a job working for the 2ⁿᵈ largest cheese factory in the country in Corona, California. The company also made pure protein from cheese. My job back then was to move 100lb sacks of protein into freight trucks. When I looked at the order forms I noticed that some of the protein sacks where going to people's houses. I asked my foreman about this one time and he told me that these people who purchased these made protein supplements out of them in their own garages and then they try to market them.

I remember saying to him, "I thought protein supplements were made in clinics and laboratories by scientists (like the magazine said)." He chuckled a bit and told me the truth that many protein supplements are made in people's garages. When they become big then they mass produce it in a factory. I will never forget what he said to me, "You don't need a doctor's degree or any degree at all to make supplements. It isn't regulated by the FDA."

The Fads

When I started weight training in the late 1980's one particular supplement was extremely popular and just about everybody in the gym was taking it, including myself, it was chromium picolante. It was hailed as a miracle supplement because it could do everything: increase muscle mass, promote fat loss, give you more energy, and some even said that it would make you virile in bed.

By the early 1990's this chromium picolante supplement seem to have fallen off from the face of the earth. Nobody talks about it anymore. Many people from my gym said that it doesn't work. That's because by then another supplement fad was in the

80

works and it was overshadowing this supplement. People were getting into yohimbi extracts and sarsaparilla. According to the advertisement, Native Americans used to take them in order to increase their hormone levels. They made themselves more muscular and strong. It supposed to make them more aggressive when it comes to doing battle. Native Americans also took them in order to increase their sex drive.

A college professor who studied Native Americans said something about the advertising he saw on muscle magazines, "I never found these aggressive, muscular, horny Indians who took these things for those reasons." Yes, some of them did eat it, but they ate it as part of their staple diet and not to develop those things that they've mentioned. Like all fads, these faded too and are no longer advertised in muscle magazines.

Of course there are more fads out there, but I just wanted to give you a few examples that existed in the past. So this way you don't make the same mistakes I did by wasting hard earn money on them. If you want to put all your eggs into one basket then put it in the *Trinitarian Principle*: training, recuperation, and proper nutrition. No need to look outside from these three. They've been around for a long time and they will certainly never fade like those fads.

Supplements that Do Work

You guys are probably still wondering if there are any supplements out there that do work. The answer to this is yes, there are some that do work. But first you must understand that supplements are just that, supplements. They will never replace what proper nutrition, hard training, and recuperation can give you. Once you have that clearly in your head then let me tell you about the ones that do work:

Multi-Vitamins and Minerals

If you eat balance meals then there would be no need for this supplement, but it's not a bad thing if you do decide to take them. Keep in mind though, if you do take in more vitamins and minerals than what your body needs then it's usually eliminated by way of urination. But fat soluble vitamins such A, D, E, and K are stored in your fat.

Since you are working out your body would slightly demand for more vitamins and minerals. All you need is a tablet a day and you're good to go. Again, no need to mega-doze, it will not make you any healthier.

Protein Meal Bars or Drinks

I mentioned this one in the protein section. Protein along with carbs and some fat is considered a meal. Use it as a snack between lunch and dinner. Just be sure though that it is a complete protein.

Creatine

It is worth it to invest on this supplement. Creatine can potentially give you increase in strength, increase in recuperation, and increase in energy. Creatine is part of the protein's building blocks (amino acid) and is found in meat and fish. Past studies done by scientists who are not associated or working for any supplement companies discovered that creatine works great for athletes who are doing anaerobic type exercises such as sprinting, power lifting, weight training, and such. An increase in progress has been seen anywhere from 5-12%. On the other hand, athletes who do long, endurance like aerobic type exercises such as long distance running, cycling, and swimming made no significant progress at all.

Creatine helps regenerate the body's ATP (Adenosine Triphosphate). ATP transport energy at cellular levels for metabolism. This is crucial when doing high level of resistance exercises such as H.I.T.

During high intensity training there are damages done to tissues or muscle fibers at a cellular level. During recuperation period creatine also promotes the increase of myonuclei, which is heavily involved in muscle fiber repair.

Some people will claim that they've gain a pound or so in one week with the use of creatine. This can be true because creatine does bind to water molecule. If you don't see any weight gains don't worry about it. In time you will.

When creatine first came out I had doubts about it, but when I started using it and my clients started using it we discovered that it works. You do have to take this with a drink that is high in sucrose or fructose so that the insulin level in your body would spike up temporarily. This would improve your body's assimilation of this supplement. Usually mixing creatine with apple juice or cranberry juice would do the trick.

Creatine has gotten a bad publicity from the media a couple of years after it was introduced as a supplement. Some people have experienced kidney problems, nausea, jitters, and even liver problems. Some have even died from it. The problem was that people didn't use this supplement properly. I believe this had something to do with how it was being taken. People were simply overloading or mega dosing on it and some were not drinking enough water.

When I first bought this supplement from a friend he told me to load up on it for 2 to 3 weeks in order to feel the full effect. This was called the *loading phase*. Afterwards, I can take it regularly. I don't remember how exactly I loaded up on it. I believe I was doing 4-5 tbsp instead of 2. But I do remember experiencing some pain at the sides of my back. I believe it was hurting my kidneys. When I stopped taking this supplement my back sides felt better. I never again went back to taking this supplement, till much later. So I don't ever recommend that you do the loading phase. Just take it according to the recommended dosage on the label.

Some of you might feel nauseated and jittery because creatine has to be taken with a sugary liquid on an empty stomach. Some of you might be sensitive to high sugar. If this is the case for you then just take creatine in its pure form by mixing it with water. Be sure to take it along with your meal instead of an empty stomach. So this way your sugar level from your meal would still go up.

If you're perfectly fine and have no issues in taking this supplement then I would recommend that you take it right after a workout. If you are not working out then I recommend that you take it early in the day, between breakfast and lunch. So this way its better utilized by your muscles.

Supplements always come and go. I'm sure by the time this book is publish there might be a couple more new supplements that are out in the market already. Be sure to do your research on them before you invest on them. Again, don't think that supplements are the answer to getting rid of your skinny self. You still have to train hard, get plenty of rest, and eat well.

CHAPTER 15

WATER

Water is far more important than food. You can survive for weeks without food, but without water you can expect to survive for only several days. Water is ever present in our body. About 60% of our bodyweight is water. Our muscle is about 70-80% water; of course the percentage would be more if your muscles are well developed.

Water has many functions in our body, which I'm not going to go over in this book. The only main thing you have to worry about is staying well hydrated. I always recommend that you drink anywhere from a gallon to a gallon and half a day. It is quite alright to go a little overboard on drinking water. You do have the luxury of peeing the excess out. Of course it might not be a luxury at all if you are in a middle of something, like being stuck on a heavy traffic.

I will never forget this lady who always comes to the gym with her little 6 year old girl. One day she spent 1 hour doing aerobics and over 1 hour doing weight training. I remember her finishing her workout and she was walking with her little 6 year old daughter who was right in front of her. All of a sudden she collapsed to the floor, right on top of her daughter. I assisted in moving her off of her daughter and helped her get up. The gym owner, Denny Kakos, brought a chair over and we had her seated on it. Denny gave her a cold sugary drink, which was Gatorade.

I remember how hot she felt when I touched her. And afterwards how cold she felt when I assisted her back on her feet again after sitting for a while. For a moment I thought she had a fever of some sort and that was the reason why she collapsed. But in later conversation I had with her she told me she was very dehydrated.

Water helps regulate your body's temperature. It is very important when you are doing strenuous exercises like weight training that you make sure you have your water close to you. Always sip it during your workouts, because you do lose a lot of water through sweat and respiration.

Never substitute juices, sodas, teas, coffee, and such for water. These liquids are not the same. Some of them can even dehydrate you. Don't be fooled by those so-called electrolyte drinks that claim to be better than water. That is not true. Nothing is better and more natural for us than water.

CHAPTER 16

A GOOD DIET

Let's go ahead and do an outline of your diet plan along with supplements. This is only a rough draft in order to give you some idea. You can change or modify this to your liking. Also adjust the servings in order to get the calories you need:

Breakfast

- 6 egg white

- ½ cup of dry Oatmeal cooked in a microwave or 2 whole wheat breads

- Fruit or 1 cup of 100% Fruit Juice (preferably orange)

- 1 tablet of multi-vitamins and minerals

Supplements

- Creatine taken with Apple Juice or Cranberry Juice. Or, you can also schedule to take this supplement right after your workout (Can be taken with a meal as well).

Lunch

- 1 cup of Rice or 1 cup of Beans or 1 Large Potato

- 6 oz. of Meat (chicken, fish, or steak)

- 4-6 oz. of Steam Vegetable

- Fruit

Snack

- Protein Meal Bar or Protein Drink (with a banana blended in)

Dinner

- 1 cup of Rice or 1 cup of Beans or 1 Large Potato

- 6 oz. of Meat (chicken, fish, or steak)

- 4-6 oz. of Steam Vegetable

- Small Salad (low sodium dressing is optional)

Snack (Optional if you need more calories)

- Yogurt or 1 tbsp. of Peanut Butter on 1 Wheat Bread or 6oz of Tuna

"Man's Proper stature is not one of mediocrity, failure, frustration, or defeat, but one of achievement, strength, and nobility. In short, man can and ought to be a hero."

--Mike Mentzer

PART III

Training Principles

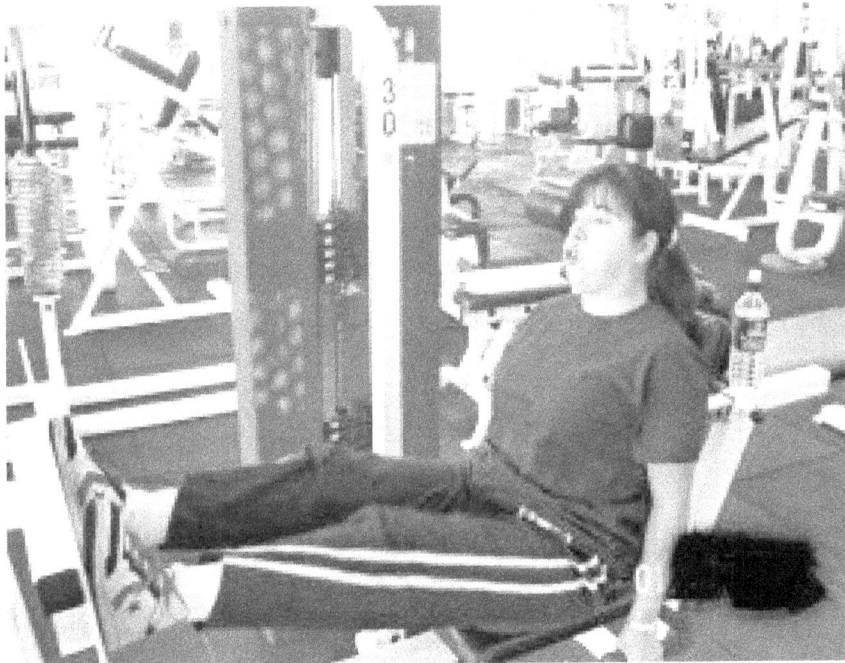

Adriana Garcia doing Leg Presses

CHAPTER 17

REPS AND SETS

Rep is a short word for *repetition.* Gym aficionados like to say *reps* when they are referring to how many times they are going to lift the weights or how many times they have lifted it. There are only 2 ways you can perform a rep in an exercise, either by pulling the resistance towards you or by pushing the resistance away from you. Examples of muscles doing the pulling motion would be your back and biceps muscles and a good example of muscles doing the pushing motion would be your chest and triceps muscles.

A set refers to a completed number of reps. For example if you are doing biceps curls with a 50lb barbell and you finished at the 10th rep then that is called a set. To say it in another way, a set is basically a collection of reps. Even if you do one rep with an exercise it is still considered a set.

Alright, reps and sets, why do people do reps and sets in the gym? In the real world we don't do reps and sets. When we lift a couch for example and move it from point A to point B we are not doing reps or sets with it. True, that couch might be heavy, but it's not going to develop your muscles in the same way as doing reps and sets with it. The reason why you don't develop large muscles when lifting a couch is because it is a static hold, meaning you are just holding it up. Now if you start doing curls or squats with that couch then you will certainly increase the size of your muscles, because this constitute work through the full range of motion of your muscles.

Our muscles were designed to contract and to extend. That design is put into application when doing weight training exercises. So when your muscles are contracting against the resistance that you are lifting up where the muscle is shortening it is referred to as a *positive lift (concentric movement)*. When you are extending the resistance down or lowering it where the muscle is lengthening that is referred to as a *negative lift (eccentric movement)*. When the resistance is at the very top of the lift it is called *peak contraction*. When the resistance is fully extended down to its starting point then that is called an *extended position*.

A typical rep scheme usually goes in this order: Extended Position →Positive Lift → Peak Contraction → Negative Lift. Just to give you a better picture, let's go back to biceps curls. You have a 50lb barbell in front of you. You picked up the weight with both of your hands and you are now holding it. This is your extended position. Once you start to curl the barbell up, you are performing the positive lift. When you reach the top of your curl you are at peak contraction. As you start lowering weight down, you are performing the negative lift. And of course it's back again at the extended position.

Proper Rep Scheme

Now that you understand what a rep scheme is you must also understand that there is an *effective* rep scheme in order to get the most stimulation out of your muscles during the exercise. If you observe how most people in the gym train you might have seen them throwing weights around when performing their reps. They may be swinging their bodies back and forth when doing biceps curls or bouncing the weight on their chest when they are doing bench presses. They are doing this in order to use more weights or

93

do more reps. This is called *cheating*. Why is it called cheating, because you are cheating your muscles from getting the full benefit from the exercise. In other words, it doesn't hit your muscles 100%. You must never develop such bad habits. This can lead to an injury in the long run. Plus, once you develop this bad habit it becomes very hard to break.

The positive lift of your rep should be performed without jerking or bouncing the weights around. You simply lift the weights in a controlled fashion at a moderate speed. When you get to the peak contraction of your rep hold it for 2 to 3 seconds before doing the negative lift. The negative lift should be moving twice as slow as when you did the positive lift. Once you've reached the extended position hold it for a second and then repeat the process again.

This proper rep scheme is indeed very difficult compare to just lifting the weights itself without paying much attention to form or speed. To me that would be a hit and miss workout, because momentum comes into play and again it becomes a cheating rep. The proper rep scheme I just described is a complete hit, because it is your muscles that are doing all the work.

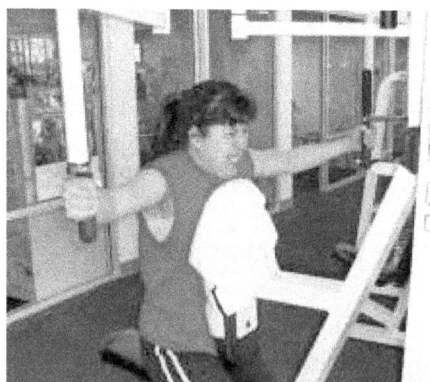

Adriana Garcia

Proper rep scheme may be difficult but it is rewarding.

CHAPTER 18

TRAINING TO POSITIVE FAILURE

If there is a key to developing muscle mass this is it. *Training to positive failure* is the most important training principle there is. This is the best way to stimulate your muscles to grow. Training to positive failure means performing the positive lift of your rep scheme to a point where you can not move the weights anymore for another rep, not even by an inch. This means that you have temporarily exhausted your muscles.

Let's go back to doing bicep curls again. Let's say you are doing barbell curls with 50lbs. You have done 3 rep curls so far and they felt rather easy. The 4th rep you start to feel your biceps fatiguing. The 5th rep you start to strain. The 6th rep felt harder to do than the 5th rep. The 7th rep you barely got the barbell up to peak contraction. The 8th rep is taking everything you got and you feel that you wouldn't be able to complete the 9th rep. You dug deep into yourself and kept going at it and you gave it everything you got and you were only able to do a half of a rep. You try again, but the barbell only moved slightly. You give it one more try, but the barbell just won't move anymore from that extended position. This is indeed a good example of training to positive failure.

You can rest assure that you have stimulated your biceps muscle 100%. With proper recuperation and nutrition you can be sure that your muscle will grow in strength and mass. To know if you are in the right path, the next time you do barbell curls and if you were able to perform 9 to 10 reps to positive failure with it instead of 8 reps that you did before then you have done it. You have gotten stronger.

There is quite a level of discomfort when performing positive failure. There's just no other way around it. You may like it or you may not, but if you truly desire to get rid of your skinny self by way of gaining muscle mass then you are going to have to perform it. In time you will get used to it and you may even like it. I, myself, have come to a point where if I don't perform positive failure it feels like I didn't get a full workout.

Some of you might fear getting an injury from doing positive failure. If your form is good throughout your set then you minimize the chances of this. It is important though that you warm up thoroughly first before you engage in training to positive failure. Warm ups will be explained later. Be sure that you don't have any pre-existing injuries before performing positive failure. Again, see a doctor and have a physical check up. Ask the doctor if it's alright for you to do strenuous exercises.

Target Rep

Target rep is about setting a number you want to achieve in your rep count so that when you are performing your exercises you are shooting for that number. Let's go back and use barbell curls again as an example: If your target rep for this exercise is 10 and you trained to positive failure and you managed to achieve 7 reps with it. Then you were 3 reps shy of your target rep. With much recuperation and proper nutrition you come back to perform this same exercise again and this time you were able to achieve 9 reps to positive failure. You were just 1 rep shy of achieving that target rep, but you are moving in positive direction because your strength has increased. Again, you took some time to recuperate and you ate well. You come back to doing the same exercise again and this time you achieved 10 reps to positive failure. Then you have done it!

You should feel proud of yourself for getting to that target rep. This is a good time now to increase the weight on that barbell curls by 5-10%. Yes, the process will start all over again as you shoot for target rep of 10.

This by the way is the best indicator as to whether or not you are making progress by getting stronger and bigger. Having a target rep to shoot for will certainly help you achieve that. Mentally, it will get you motivated in the gym as you strive for it. You go in to the gym knowing what you need to do and what you want to accomplish.

The number you want to achieve as your target rep is up to you. I always recommend and set my target rep at 8 for all my exercises, including abs and legs. Some of the clients I've trained prefer 10 or 12. I don't recommend you go any higher than 12. Because if you do, you'll more likely to be challenged by your cardio capacity, especially on legs, and also lactic acid will build up and you might prematurely go into positive failure because of it. If you set it any lower than 8 then you might find out that you are not working the muscles enough for proper stimulation.

The exercises that you are going to be doing in my book I would recommend a target rep of 8. Later on when you become familiar with the exercises and feel that you want to change the setting of your target rep you can do so. But for now stick with 8.

CHAPTER 19

PROPER FORM

Proper form is something I can never emphasize enough. Proper form is not only effective in targeting the muscles themselves, but it's also effective in minimizing potential injuries. I don't ever recommend that you pay attention to how most of the people in the gym are training these days. Many of them train in very sloppy ways anyway. They *cheat* their reps just so they could lift more weights and/or in order to do more reps. Again, performing your reps in such a haphazard way could lead to potential injuries in the long run.

Remember, once you've injured something. The chance of you re-injuring that same area again is very likely. So pay attention to your form and never allow yourself to get sloppy. Though I know that there is a temptation to cheat your reps during your set so that you could achieve your target rep, don't. Though I can never promise you that you will never get injured from doing your exercises in a proper form, I can certainly promise you that it is less likely to happen.

Full Range of Motion

Upon reading proper rep scheme you may have gotten the hint as to how important full range of motion is. In order to work the muscles to the fullest you have to do full range of motion. This means during the exercise you extend the muscle you are working on as far as your joints will allow you too and to bring it up all the way to peak contraction where your joints will not allow anymore movement.

As of late, many bodybuilders in the gym are doing partial reps. This seems to be a trend that the so-called pro-bodybuilders who are heavily taking steroids have started doing. The reason for this is just so they could lift heavy weights. For you who plan on training naturally, don't fall for this type of bad habit. You will develop better and fuller muscles through full range of motion.

Not How Much You Can Lift, But How You Lift It

Back then I thought I had to lift a certain amount of weight in order to get rid of my skinny self. I thought I had to bench press over 300lbs, squat 500lbs, and curl 135lbs in order to be muscular. Sure lifting heavy weights will add more density to your muscles, but how you lift the weights count more.

I remember Hector from my gym. He's a medium size person who stands about 5'7" and weighs 170lbs. He always impresses the guys in the gym, including myself, with his feats of strength. He could bench press 405lbs for 6 reps, do 1000lbs of leg presses for 8 reps, and do 300lbs of the wide pulldowns for 6 reps.

Then there's another guy in my gym by the name of Allen. He too stands at 5'7" and weighs about 185lbs. Allen is far more muscular than Hector. As a matter of fact he had a number of 1st place wins in some of the natural bodybuilding contests he entered. When it comes to training, Allen doesn't use as much weight as Hector does. The most I've seen Allen do on a bench press was 225lbs and 500lbs on the leg press. But what makes him more muscular than Hector was his form. Each of his reps is executed slowly and perfectly in full range of motion. Hector on the other hand cheats his reps by moving fast and doing only partial reps.

Allen once told me that he's a perfectionist by nature. It truly reflected on his physique and on his workouts. To top it off, Allen is almost 20 years older than Hector and he had never once been side tracked by an injury. While Hector, on the other hand, has had some injuries that forced him to take long lay-offs from training. So it's always better to be safe if you plan on doing this for the rest of your life.

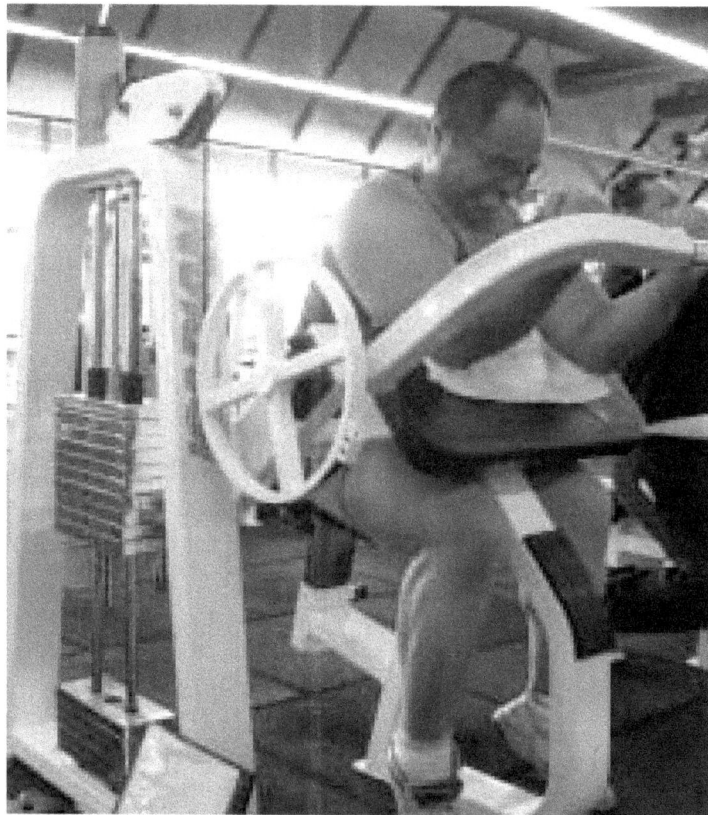

Full Range of Motion gives the muscles more work for better result.

PART IV

Exercises

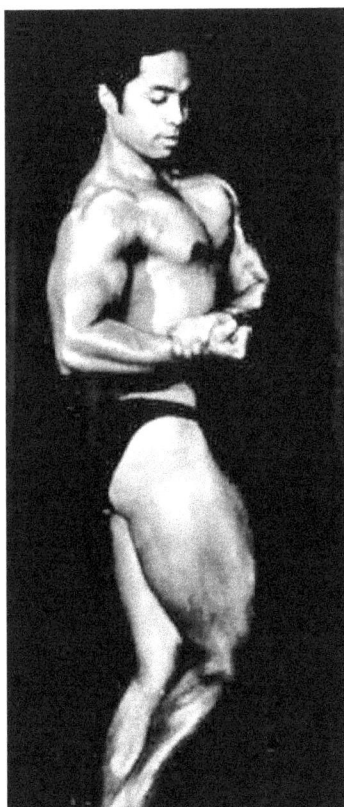

CHAPTER 20

EXERCISES

There are a lot of resistance exercises that you can do for specific body parts. No longer is resistance exercises reserved to just dumbbells and barbells. Technology has certainly brought forth different array of exercise equipments. Different gyms tend to offer different exercise equipments. No two gyms are ever alike. So the exercises I'm describing in this book are the most common ones that you, as a bodybuilder, can do at just about any gym. Of course you are always welcome to substitute any exercises you want, given that you perform them in a proper way.

Those of you who decided to workout at home can get an effective workout by making sure that you have the equipment to workout different body parts. Just be sure that you don't outgrow the weights you use. Continue to invest on equipments that will give variety to your home workouts.

Compound and Isolation Movement

Compound and isolation movement will be mentioned quite a bit on the exercises that I'm going to describe. Just to touch up on what these terms mean:

Isolation exercises usually refer to a single joint movement that small muscle groups such as biceps, triceps, calves, and so on usually perform. Isolation exercises can also be performed on large muscle groups such as legs, chest, back and shoulders.

Compound exercises usually refer to multiple joint movements. They involve not just the target muscle, but other smaller muscle groups as well. For example if you're doing bench press to workout your chest, even though the chest muscle is the main target you are also involving triceps, shoulders, and forearms in the process.

Calves

Calf muscles, also known as *gastranemous*, are located at the back of your legs, between the knees and ankles. If you want to see them fully flexed turn your back to a full length mirror. Turn your head around as far back as you can and look down between your knees and ankles. Stand on your tip toes and watch the bulges come out. Pound per pound the calf muscles are the strongest muscles in your body. They are highly resistant to fatigue and they are the fastest muscles to recuperate.

Many bodybuilders complain that their calf muscles don't respond well to resistant training or as good as the rest of their body parts. As a personal trainer I have discovered that the calf muscles are the most neglected body parts among the bodybuilders or trainers. Those that do train them are not training them as hard as the rest of the body parts. You will often see them doing high repetition and high sets.

High reps and high sets will more likely do nothing for your calves. As I mentioned that calf muscles are highly resistant to fatigue and they are the fastest recuperating muscles. So doing high reps and high sets would be a natural thing for them. What they need is a good H.I.T. You are better off stimulating them with one intense set of a target rep of 8 done to positive failure.

Standing Calf Machine

Get underneath the shoulder pads. Place the balls of your feet on the block. Stand erect on the machine with your knees locked. Be sure your toes are pointing straight forward. Bring your heels down as far as they could possibly go and then raised them up as high as you possibly can. Be sure to follow the proper rep scheme and train to positive failure.

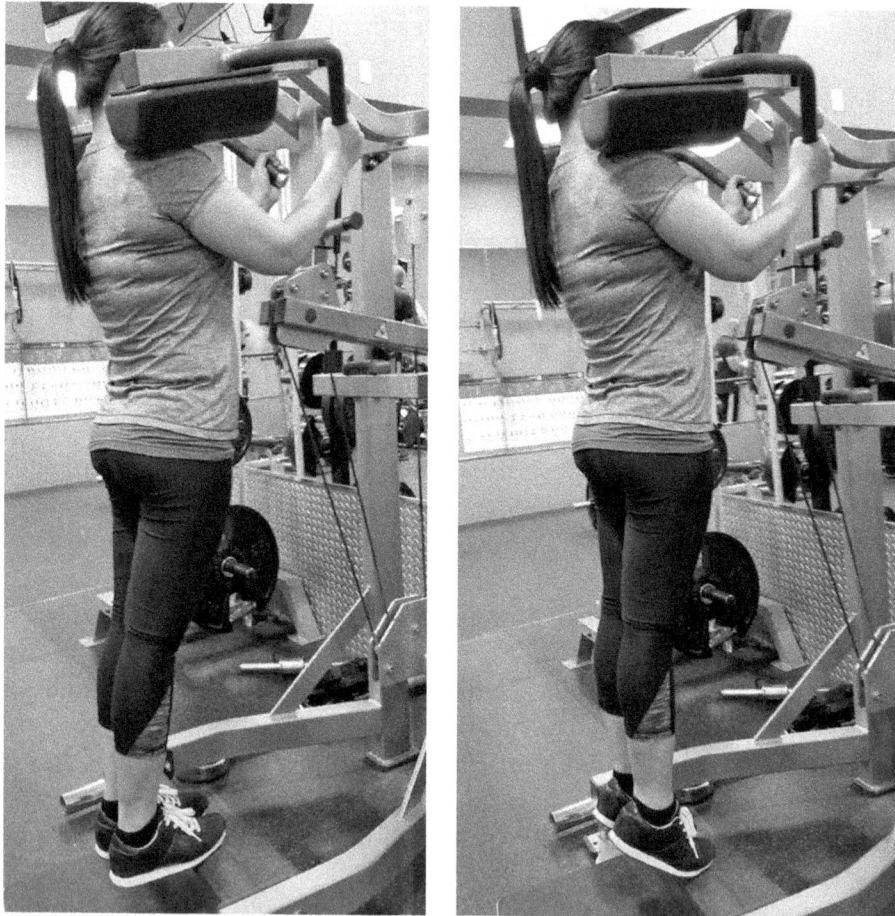

Shiela Garcia

Seated Calf Raises

If standing calf raises bothers your knees then seated calf raises will help alleviate that. Sit on the machine. Place the pads close to your knees. Do not place the pads very close to your knees or on top of it, you run the risk of it slipping off and possibly hurting yourself. Just to play it safe, place the grip of your hands on top of the pads. This will help ensure that it doesn't slip off. But do not use your grip to help with your lifts. Use the same feet position and training procedure as standing calf raises.

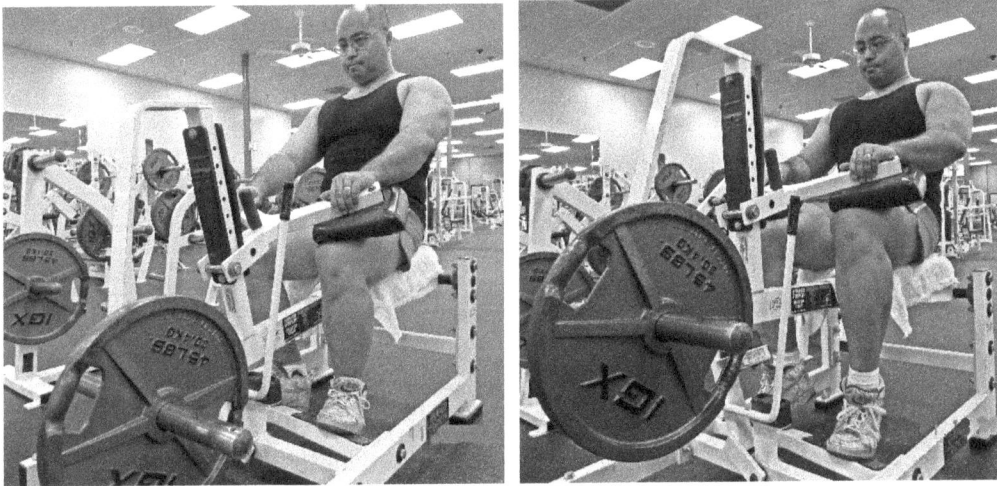

Thighs

Thighs are often times referred to as quadriceps or quads. They are the largest and most powerful muscles in your body. Thigh muscles are the most demanding muscles in your body when it comes to workouts. They can take a great deal amount of energy from you and they can also put your cardiovascular system to the test. So don't feel weird if you feel drained and out of breath after working them out.

Believe it or not, since they are so demanding to your system there are some bodybuilders out there that would rather skip training them. If you ever see a huge bodybuilder with a big upper body wearing baggy pants chances are they are hiding their puny legs.

"Oh man, I got legs today." You may hear bodybuilders saying this often in the gym. But seriously, there really should be no reason at all for skipping legs. There's so much to gain from them, because they are not only beneficial to your lower body and cardio, but also to your upper body.

There are some scientific facts, although not yet fully confirmed, that working out your thigh muscles hard can actually release your natural growth hormones throughout your body. So in other words, the hard workout from them can have a synergistic effect on your other muscles. Hormones can truly affect muscle mass and strength.

In my own personal experience I find this to be true. Back then when I first started training I was only interested in developing my chest and biceps. Other body parts didn't matter as much to me. Sure my chest and biceps did develop, but not much.

When I started training legs just as hard my chest and biceps developed even more. The body works in a systematic way. So never skip or even dread doing your legs.

Squats

For those of you who have not done this type of compound exercise before it would take quite a bit of practice. Why, because if this exercise is not done properly it can potentially lead to some injuries, particularly to your lower back and knees. Once you've mastered this movement then you'll see that this is the best exercise you could ever do for your quads.

So if this is new to you, then I recommend you start off with no weights on the bar for now. For safety be sure to always do this exercise inside a squat rack and not outside. Adjust the safety bars inside to your proper level. So when you go to positive failure those safety bars will take the weight off from you.

Now let's begin. Place the bar at the bottom back part of your neck and have it rested on your shoulders. If the weight of the barbell bothers your shoulders and neck then wrap the part of the barbell that touches them with a thick towel. This will help cushion it. Once you are standing with the barbell on your shoulders, spread your legs apart to about shoulder width. There should be a slight outward angle to your feet where your toes are pointing out. Arch your lower back and have your head facing slightly upward. With your form this way, go ahead and start bending your knees slowly. You are now doing the negative lift of this exercise. See how far down you can go. Once you've hit the extended position hold it for a second and then do your positive lift.

There's no peak contraction to this exercise, so once you've reached the top position hold it for a second or two in order to take a breath and repeat your rep cycle.

There are a couple of things you need to know about squats. I don't advice you to lock your knees at the top position because of the way the weight is positioned on your body. You might end up with a knee problem in the future. Note too as you go down with this exercise you might have a tendency of leaning too forward, especially if you're a tall person. This is your body's way of balancing itself. But always remember to keep your back arch and your head up. Don't force yourself to go all the way down if your knees and lower back is not up to it. In time your flexibility will improve and you will be able to go all the way down. Yes, the fuller the range of motion the better you'll develop your thighs, but safety must come first.

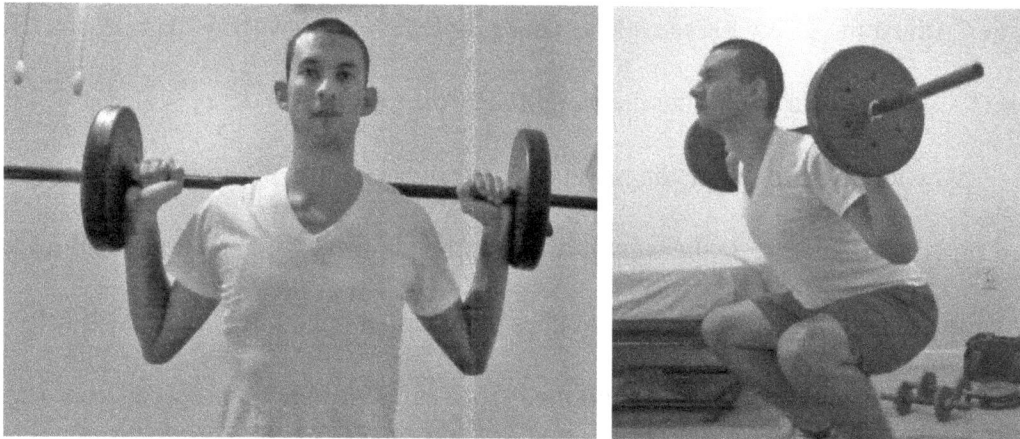

Jaime Augusto Barrientos Jr.

Leg Press

Like squats, leg press is another compound exercise that is very effective for the thigh muscles. Lie down with your back on the pad. Place your feet about a shoulder width apart. Lower the weights till your knees are almost next to your chest. Hold for a second at this extended position and then do the positive lift.

Leg press is a type of exercise that's particularly very risky to go to positive failure on. You mustn't go all the way to positive failure on your own because you'll end up stuck at the bottom, even if it has a safety feature. What I would advise you do is get close to positive failure. If you have a training partner, he or she can help you put the weight back in a safety position. If not then you can try and use your hands. When you feel close to positive failure place your hands close to your knees and push up till the weight is at the safety position so you can lock the weights at the top.

Like squats, you shouldn't lock your knees at the top position. Locking your knees may cause knee problems in the future. Again, just like squats, there's no peak contraction to this exercise.

Many trainers do not go all the way down on leg press. You can tell by how far their feet travel down. If you have a tape measure you'll see that they only go down by a foot difference. There's a couple of reason why they do this. One of them is just so they could lift more weights. Second one might be because they are not flexible enough, which they should work on improving. And the third one might be because they have their feet placed closer together on the block. Having the feet placed closer together will get blocked by upper body as you go down and the thighs won't be able to go all the way down.

Your goal with this exercise is to go down as far as you possibly can. Short movement or partial movements will not help you develop fuller, muscular thighs. Remember, the more range of motion the better your muscles will develop.

Plate Loaded Leg Press Machine

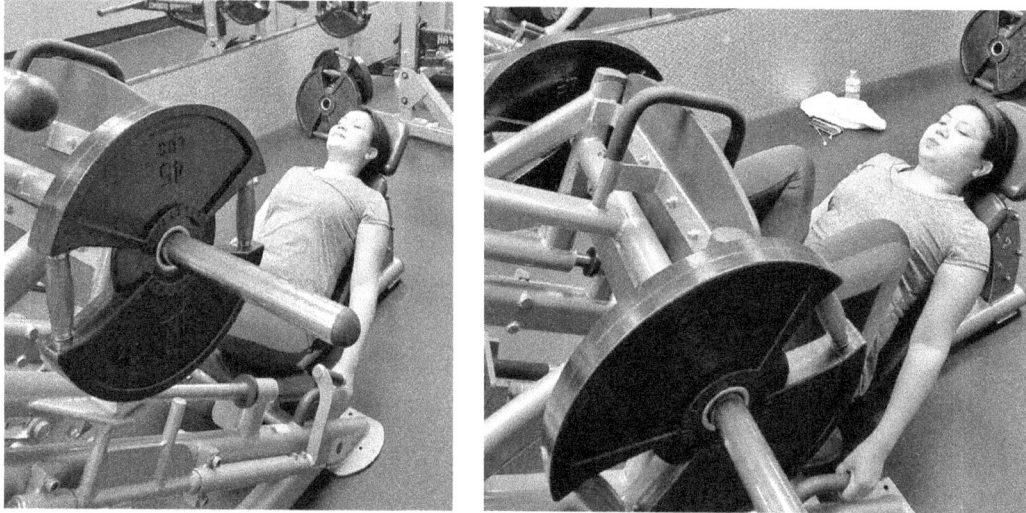

Shiela Garcia

Horizontal Leg Press Machine

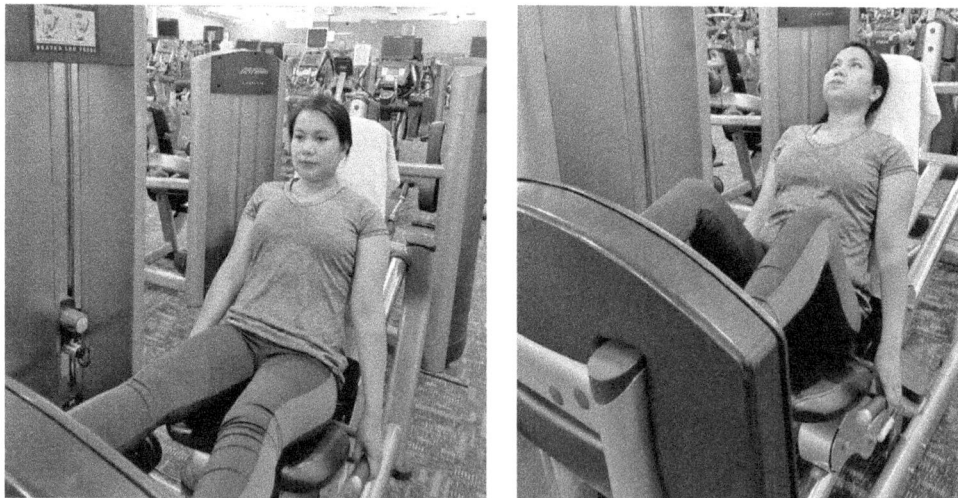

Shiela Garcia

Leg Extension

This isolation exercise truly targets just the thigh muscles as oppose to getting the hamstrings, glutes, and calves involved in the compound exercises. Sit on the seat. Have your feet go under the pad. Be sure the pad is very close to your feet and not so much on your shin. Do a couple of reps with light weights just to be sure that your leg movement is smooth, if not then make the proper adjustments.

From an extended position go ahead and lift the weights till your legs are at peak contraction. It's alright to lock your knees on this one. If you experience pain at this lock position then there is something wrong with your knees. Have it checked by your doctor before proceeding with this exercise or any leg exercises. Hold for two seconds at peak contraction position and then lower it slowly back down to an extended position. Repeat the cycle till you hit positive failure.

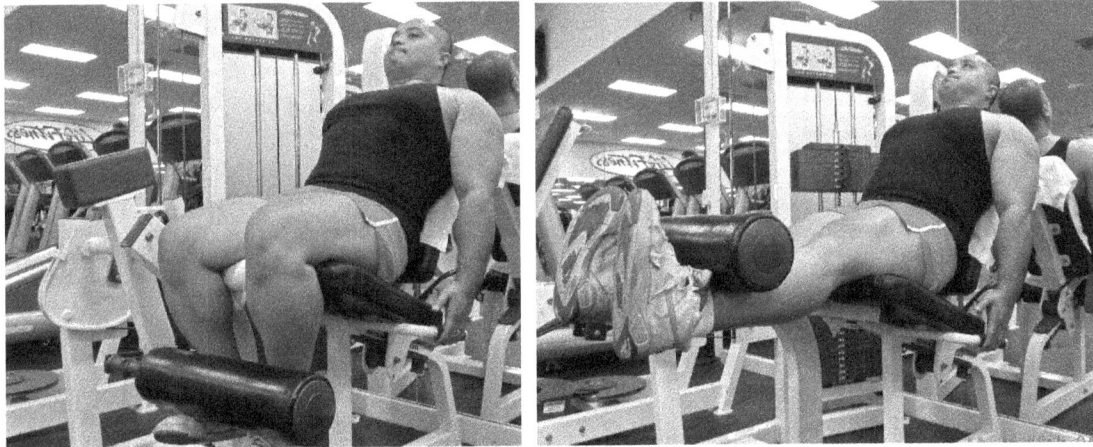

Hamstrings

These muscles are located at the opposite side of your thighs, between your buttocks or glutes and your calves. Its main function is to curl your legs. This is sort of like the biceps of your leg muscles by way it is flexed and worked out. Synergistically, hamstrings do get some work out every time you do compound exercises such as squats and leg presses. A good direct exercise for them would be the leg curls.

Leg Curls

This type of exercise can either be done lying down or seated. It just depends on which machine you prefer to use or you can alternate. Seated leg curls is easier on your lower back, but it doesn't indirectly hit the gluteus muscles like lying leg curls does. Lying leg curls are the most popular exercise for the hamstrings and most gyms have them, whereas seated leg curls tend to be not available in some gyms. But which ever one you use both of them will do the job nicely.

When you do your leg curls try to imagine that you are trying to have your heels touch your buttocks, which probably won't happen, but try to bring it up as far back as you can. At peak contraction hold it for 2 seconds and then lower it slowly back to a fully extended position. Your legs at this point should be straight. Repeat the exercise by lifting it in a control fashion.

Don't be afraid to go to positive failure. I say this because some people are afraid to go to positive failure on their hamstrings due to the burning feeling or sometimes the feeling that they are going to snap. Don't worry, it's just the immediate build up of lactic acid (metabolic waste produced by anaerobic workout). As long as the exercise is done in a proper form and proper rep scheme it is quite safe to go to positive failure for your hamstring. But do take precaution. If it gets too intense to move then stop immediately. There might be too much lactic acid and they can certainly hurt or you might have a preexisting condition.

Lying Leg Curls

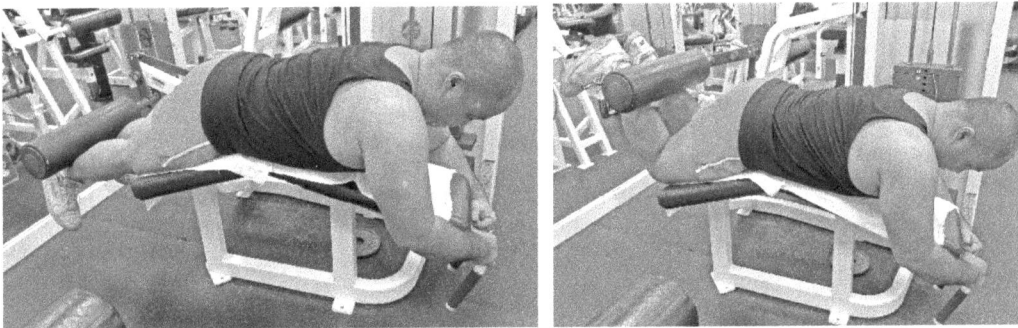

Seated Leg Curls

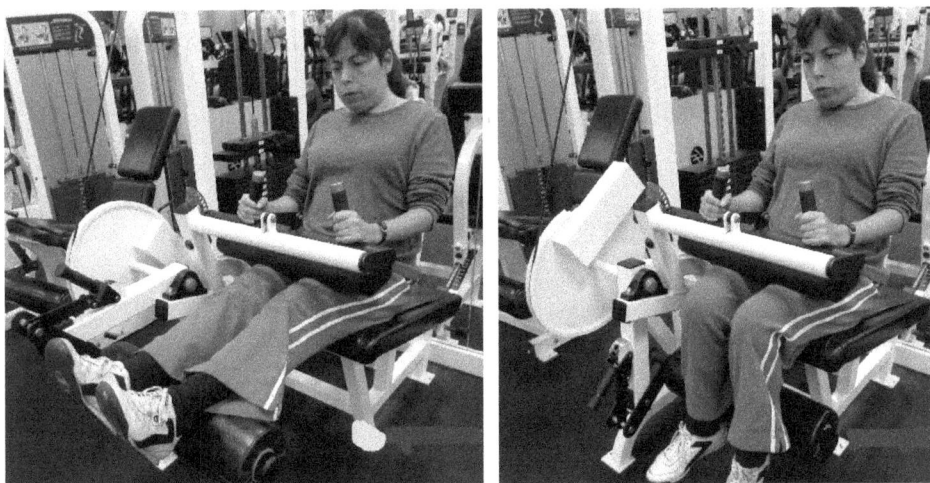

Adriana Garcia

Chest

Every man wants a well developed chest that bulges every time they wear a T-shirt. Since ancient times in Greece and Rome most of their male statues have been depicted with well developed chest. It represents power and strength. When I first started doing bodybuilding it was the chest muscles that I wanted to develop the most. I actually did more exercises for my chest than for any of my other body parts. I was so obsessed with it that I measured the circumference of my chest on a daily basis. Of course I later learned that I have to develop my back muscles as well in order to increase the circumference.

Chest is sometimes referred to as pectoral muscles. Its main function is to move your arms across your body. It helps you push objects that are in front of you. It also helps stabilize your arms when you are holding something steady. Pound per pound, your chest muscles are one of the strongest body parts in your upper body region. If the exercises for your chest are done right they do develop rather easily on most men. For women it does tend to take a bit more time. It's a very rewarding experience to watch them grow as you look at them in the mirror.

Bench Press

Most bodybuilders with big chest will tell you that they do lots and lots of bench presses in order to develop a huge chest. They fail to tell you that they also do flys or crossovers on top of that exercise.

Bench Press is indeed an excellent exercise for the chest muscles, but it is by no means the best. Bench presses involves too many muscles that can fail or get exhausted first before your chest does, such as the triceps muscle or the anterior deltoids of your shoulders (front part of your shoulders). It's not unusual at all for trainers to feel that they've worked out their shoulders or triceps more so than they've worked out their chest. A number of my clients have experienced this and so have I. In time your involved muscles will develop and you'll feel the exercise hitting your chest muscles more directly.

The way to start with the bench press exercise is to lie down on the bench with your feet spread out and flat on the floor. Your lower back should be raised up and not touching the bench at all. Your upper back should be flat on the bench.

To be safe start off with an empty Olympic bar in order to get the proper feel for the exercise. The Olympic bar weighs about 45lbs. Place your hands on the bar that is slightly wider than your shoulder width. Be sure your hands are equally spaced so that the bar is well balanced during your lifts. Lower the bar at an extended position. The bar should be slightly above your nipples. Your forearms at this position should be perfectly perpendicular to the floor. If it isn't then adjust your hand positions. Hold for a second and then lift it off your chest. Once you have gotten the feel for it and your form is perfect, go ahead and add the weights to it.

With bench press you do need a training partner in order to make sure that you safely go to positive failure. If a training partner is not available then I suggest you use a free bench (a bench that is not bolted to the floor) and do the exercise inside of a squat rack with the safety support bars set. If this is also not available then I suggest doing machine bench press. They are just as effective and much safer too.

Never do single max rep. Trainers sometimes like to test their strength on the bench press by doing single max rep. This is often performed in a haphazard way. Trainers bounce the weight on their chest and they lift their butts off the bench, just to achieve one rep. This is not effective at all in developing your chest or strength. You only run the risk of seriously injuring yourself.

Barbell Bench Press

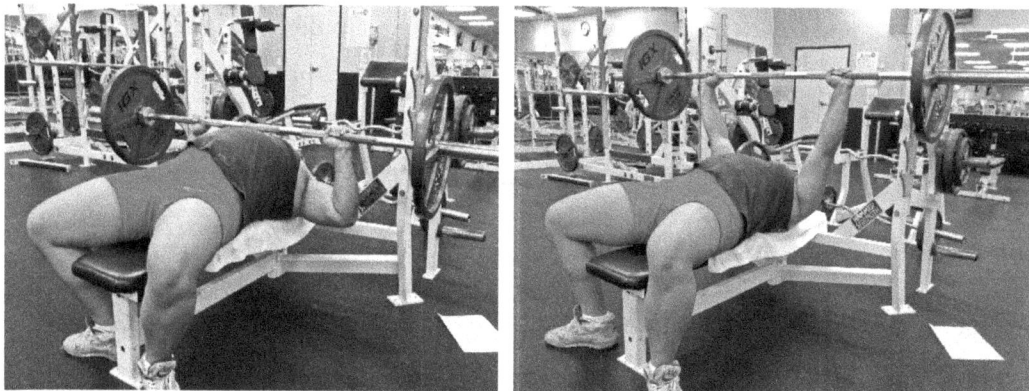

Machine Bench Press

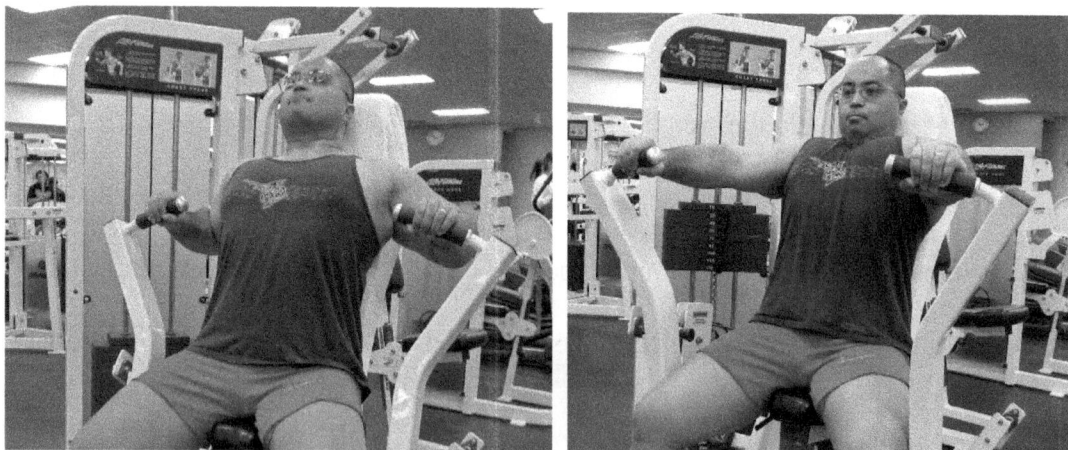

Hammer Press

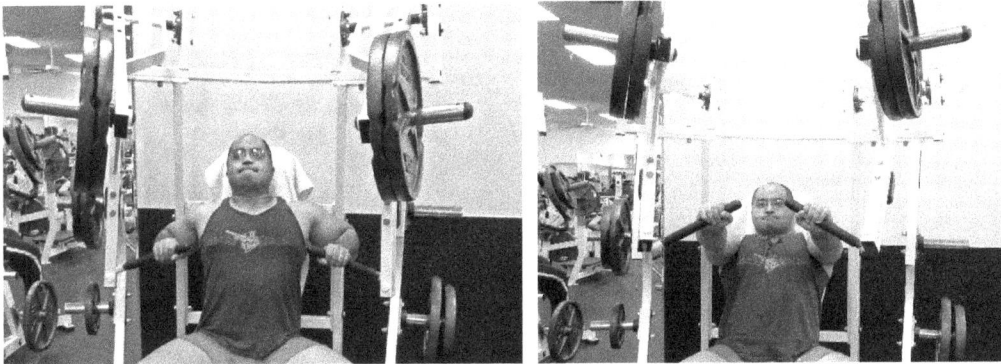

Incline Bench Press

This particular exercise is similar to bench press, except the emphasis shifts more to the upper regions of the chest. When doing this exercise be sure that you are lying on a bench that is either at a 45 or 65 degree angle. Anything higher than that then the emphasis of the exercise would shift more to the shoulder region.

When lying on the bench be sure that your lower back is arch and not touching the bench. Again, start the exercise with no weights at all on the Olympic bar. Place your hands on it slightly wider than your shoulder width. Lift the bar off and place it at the top region of your chest. At the extended position adjust your grip if necessary so that your forearms are perpendicular to the floor. Do several reps in order to get the feel for it and to understand the proper form. When you feel that you're ready go ahead and add the weights.

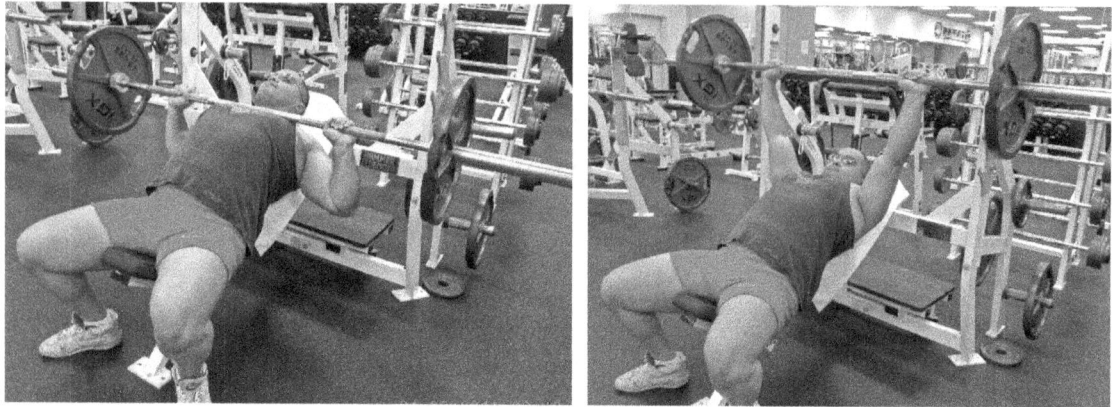

Flys

Flys are truly the best workout you could do for your chest. It hits them more directly. Flys are either done with dumbbells, cables, or machine. Which ever one you decide on the form must always remain the same. Bend your arms slightly so that you don't put too much stress on the biceps muscle. Extend your arms as far back as you possibly can in order to get a fuller range of motion and lift from there. Except for pec deck machines, where the forearms are rested against the pads. Pec Deck machines are the best chest isolation there is. It targets the chest more completely. If your gym has this, use it.

Cable Crossovers

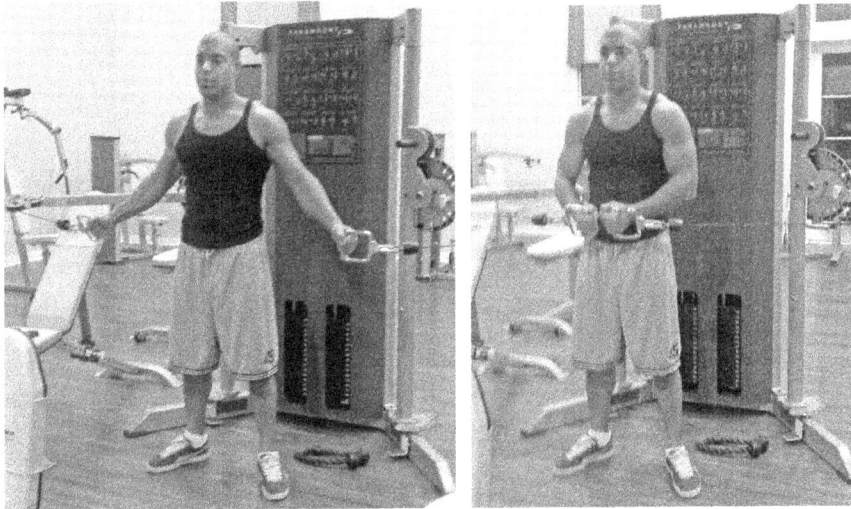

Jarrod Bryant

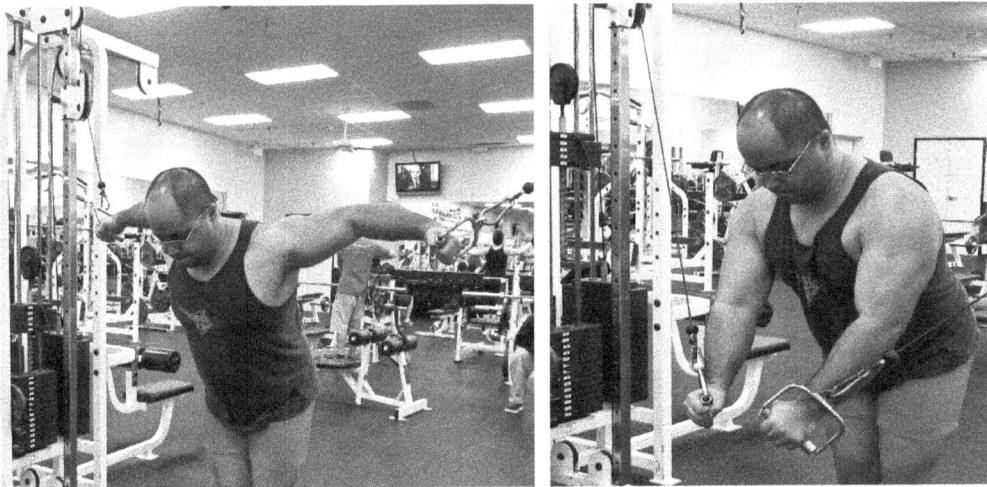

You can either pull from the middle of the cables or up.

Pec Deck

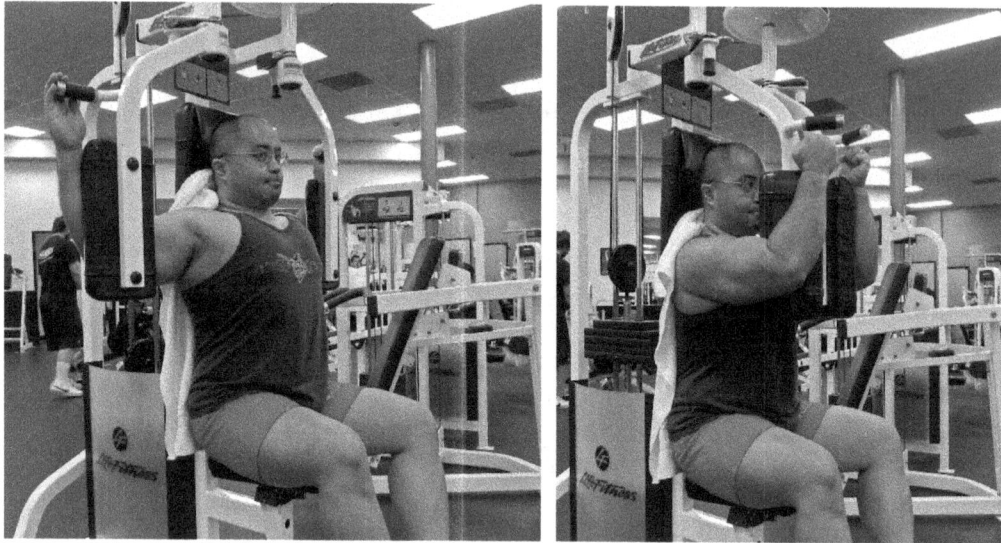

Dumbbell Flys

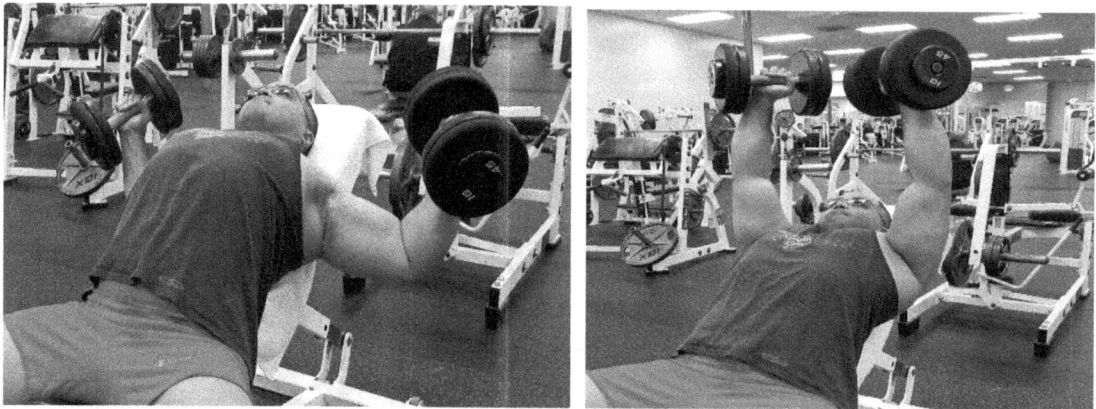

This can either be done on incline or flat bench.

Back

As you already know that the function of the back is the opposite of the chest. Chest muscles are meant for pushing objects away from your body, while the back muscles are meant for pulling the objects toward you. The back muscles are the largest muscles in your upper body. It is also the most difficult muscles to develop.

I've been to a lot of natural bodybuilding contest (drugfree) and I've seen many competitors with underdeveloped back. Even the clients I've trained and myself included have had a hard time developing the back muscles. For years I've tried figuring this out, until I've discovered a couple of things. I've discovered that we were using too much biceps into the movement and there was a lack of shoulder movement.

Unfortunately biceps comes into play at almost all of the back exercises. Biceps are a weak link. They tend to fail first before the back muscles do. The best solution is to minimize them by not contracting them too much at peak contraction. This will be explained as I describe the exercises. Along with biceps I will also explain why shoulders must come into play in order to have an effective back workout.

As with most exercises it is very important that you arch your back. This means having your upper back straight with a curve on your lower back. This will help target the upper back more during the exercises and help minimize or prevent back injury.

Wide Pulldowns

This is done with a straight bar connected to an upper cable. Sit on a padded seat with your thighs secured under the pads so that you're steady. Arch your lower back and move your head slightly forward. Grab the bar wider than shoulder width. For a starting point, allow your arms to be stretched out along with your shoulders. Imagine your shoulders almost touching your ears. Now you can either pull it down in front of your face or to the back of your head. Once you are bringing it down your arms and shoulders should be going down simultaneously. Bring it down to a point where your upper arms are slightly below parallel from the floor. Remember, if you go any lower than this the exercise will shift from your back to your biceps.

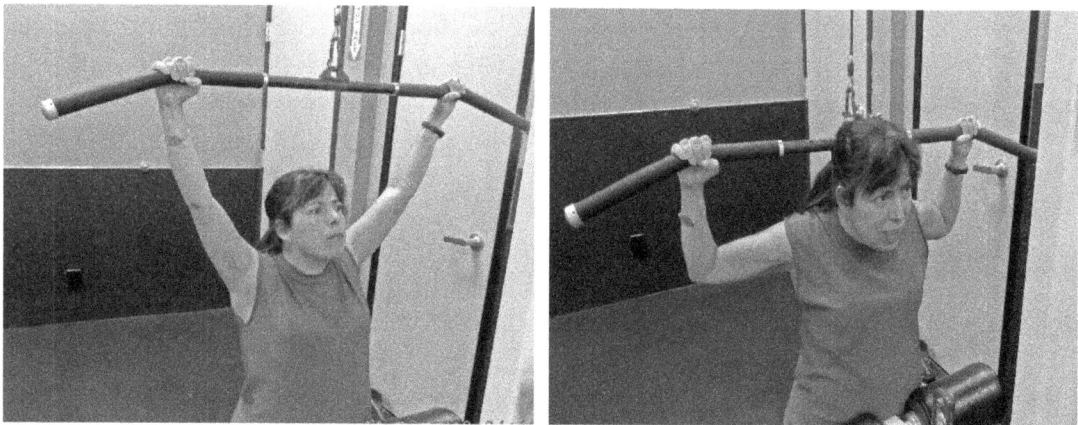

Adriana Garcia

Seated Rows

There are different variations of doing Seated Rows. They are either done with cables or with machines. Whichever one you do the principle of executing it is still the same. One thing you must never do with this exercise, never swing your upper body back and forth like a pendulum. You run the risk of injuring your lower back in the long run.

Sit on the padded seat again with your back arch. Grab hold of the V type bar. Your arms should be fully extended with your shoulders rolled forward. Your feet and legs should be fully supported in order to keep yourself steady. Your knees should be bent slightly. Your shoulders should be moving in unison with your arms. Bring the V type bar to your stomach. Avoid your elbows from going all the way back. You don't want the emphasis to shift to your biceps.

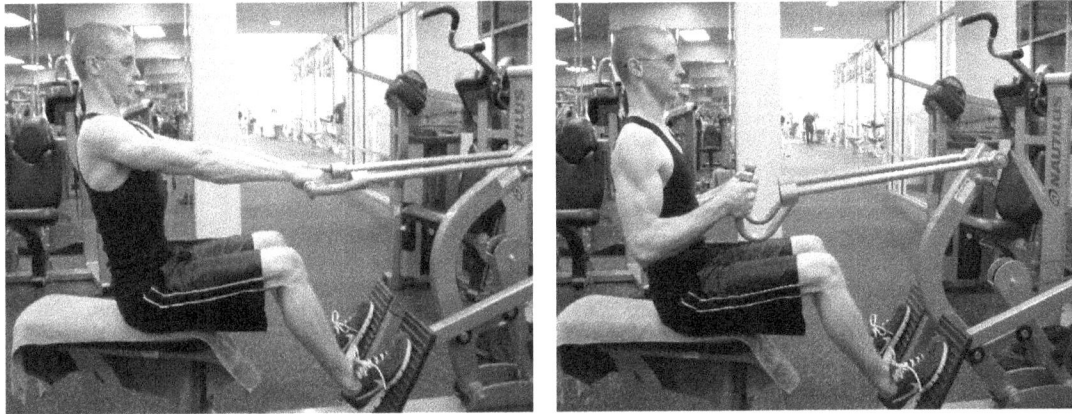

Kyle Babb

Seated Rows done on a Nautilus Machine.

Dumbbell Rows

You are going to need one dumbbell and a free bench with this particular exercise. Starting with your right side, or left side whichever you prefer, place your left knee and your left hand on the free bench. Your upper body should be parallel to the floor with your lower back arched. Now grab the dumbbell with your right hand. Again be sure your right shoulder is extended down along with your arm. Pull the dumbbell up till your upper arm is parallel to the floor. Again, your shoulder should be moving in unison with your arm. Hold for two seconds and bring it back down. Do a complete set to positive failure and do the same to the other side.

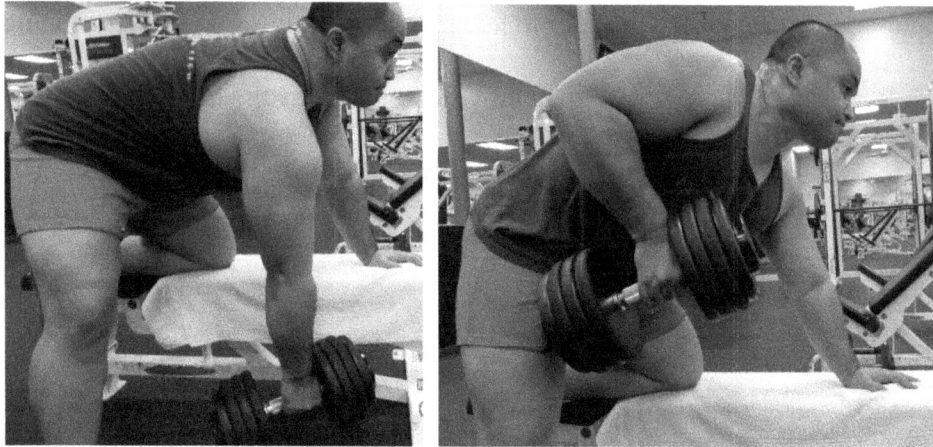

Pullovers

This particular exercise truly concentrates on the back and it doesn't involve the use of biceps. If you have a Nautilus Pullover in your gym I highly recommend that you use that. If you don't know how to use it have a personal trainer there show you how. If you don't have a Nautilus Pullover then the next best thing is to either use a cable or a dumbbell.

Using a straight bar that's attached to an upper cable, stand a couple of feet away in front of it. Grab hold of the straight bar at a shoulder width with your arms straight. Your elbows should be pointing outward and slightly down. Keep your upper body straight with your lower back arch. Bend slightly forward and bend slightly at the knees. Pull the straight bar and bring it towards your hip. Your arms range of motion should be moving slightly more than 90 degrees.

Doing pullovers with the dumbbell is different. Lie at the side of the bench with only your upper back touching it. Bring your buttocks down. Grab hold of the dumbbell with both of your hands and have your arms straight in front of you with your elbows bend slightly. This will be your starting point. Now keeping your arms steady bring the dumbbell as far back as you possibly can. From that extended position lift it back up. There's no peak contraction to this exercise so as you get it back to the top start negative lift again. Don't feel strange if you feel your ribs being stretched out. This is normal and it is an excellent exercise for expanding your rib cage.

Cable Pullovers

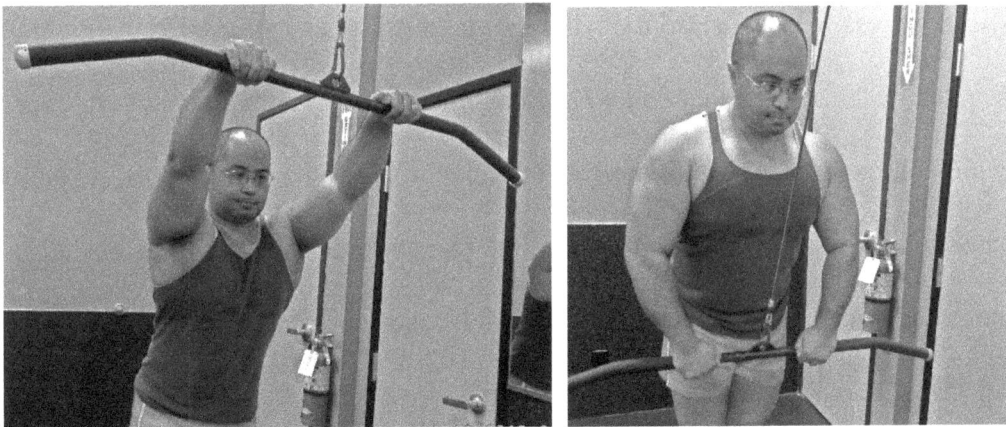

Dumbbell Pullovers

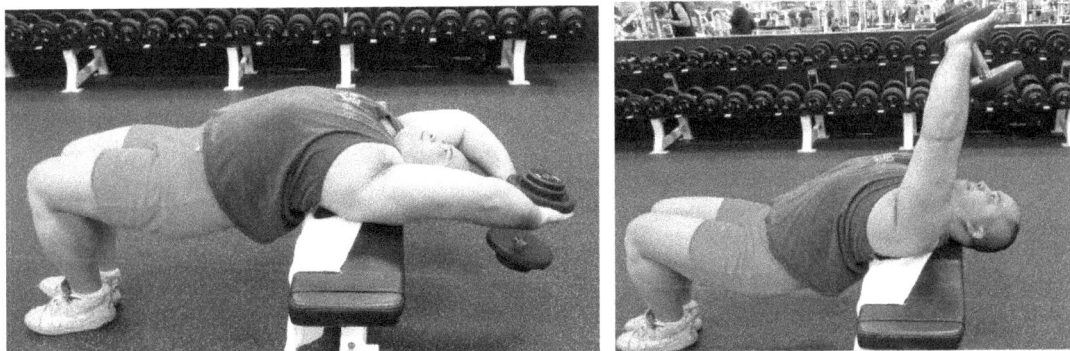

Shoulders

Shoulders are very much involved in just about any exercise that you do for your upper body. Meaning if you are doing the chest the trapezoids or traps (muscles that are connected to you neck and shoulders), front and side deltoids (muscles at the sides of your shoulder) are involved. If you are doing the back the rear deltoids, traps and rhomboid (at the center of the back) are involved. If you are either doing triceps or biceps the shoulders come in as stabilizer muscles. So it's not at all uncommon to overtrain these muscles.

There are various exercises you can do to directly target the shoulder muscles. Military press will hit the front of your deltoid muscles and your traps. Upright rows will hit more of the side of your deltoid muscles and put more emphasis on your traps. Dumbbell lateral flys will hit more of the center of your deltoids along and your traps, dumbbell posterior flys will hit more of the rear deltoids and your traps as well as rhomboid, while dumbbell anterior flys will hit more of the front deltoids with your traps. All these exercises will be described in detail.

Just like the back exercises you also have to arch your lower back on the shoulder exercises. Again, this is just to prevent and or minimize lower back injuries. Rotor cuff injury is a very common injury to shoulders. This is due to their wear and tear, as I mentioned the shoulder muscles get overtrained easily from direct and indirect exercises. Like the rest of the muscles you must give them sufficient amount of rest in order for them to improve.

Military Presses

You can perform this exercise with either barbell or machine. Whichever one you decide on just be sure you are sitting down on a seat with a padded back rest in order to support your back and to keep your upper body stable. If you are doing this with a barbell then be sure to have a partner in order to avoid getting stuck when you hit positive failure. If you don't have a partner, then perform this exercise inside a squat rack with a free bench that has a reclining capability. Adjust the safety support bars so that when you go to positive failure you can just drop the barbell on it.

Place your hands on the bar wider than your shoulder width. Be sure to have your lower back arched with your upper back against the back rest. Have your head tilted slightly forward. Lift the bar in a controlled manner. Hold at peak contraction and be sure not to lock your elbows. Lower it slowly to an extended position and have the bar go behind your head. Your forearms at this point should be perpendicular to the floor. You don't need to lower it all the way down below your neck where your mid-forearms and biceps are touching. You don't want too much triceps to come into play. The triceps are a weak part in this exercise and you don't want them to fail first. You can also do this at the front with your head back and barbell goes down in front of you.

Military Press Done at Front

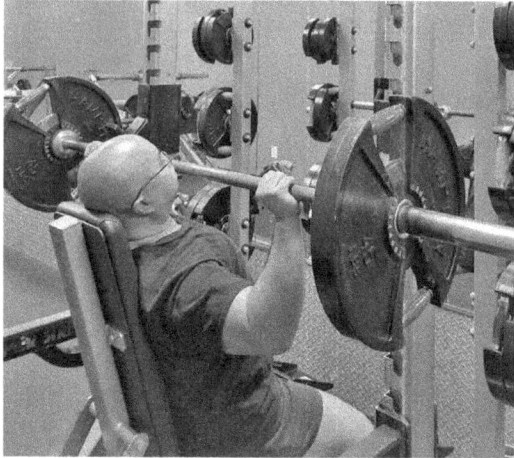

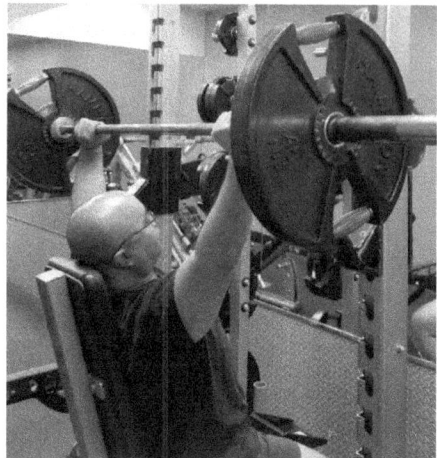

Military Press Done at the Back

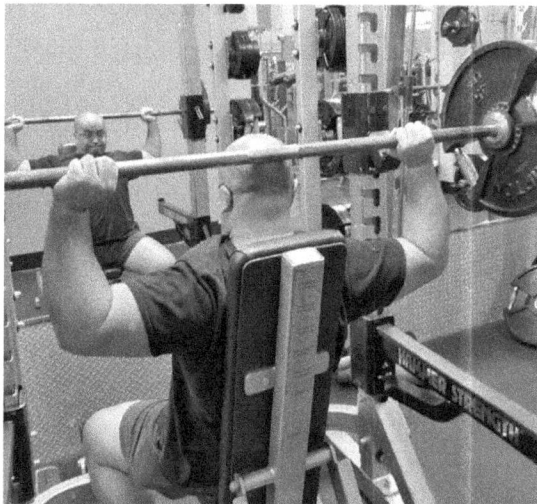

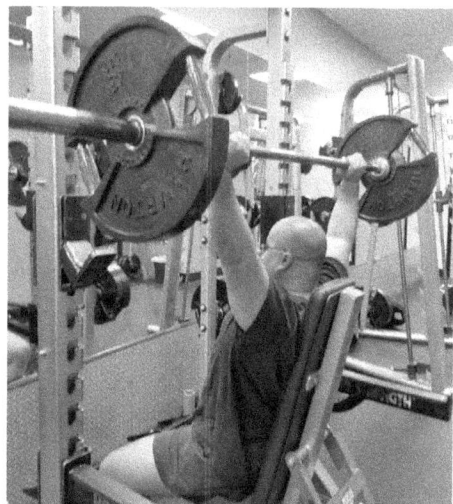

Machine Military Press

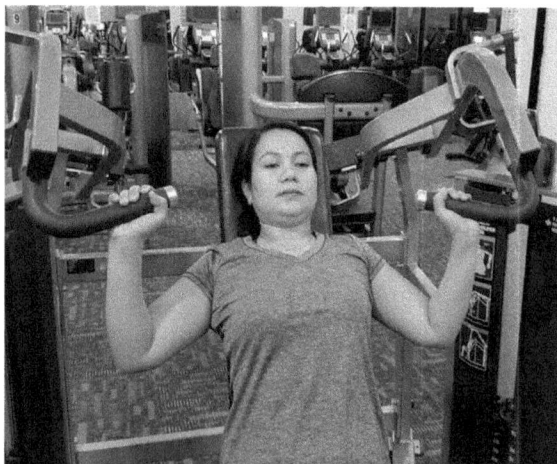

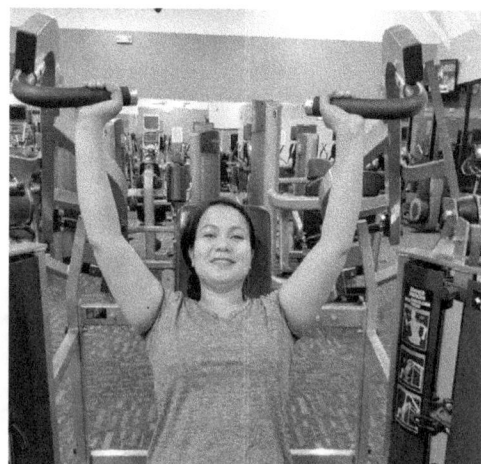

Upright Rows

This exercise can either be done by using a barbell or cable. Stand straight with your back arch and with your head slightly titled up. Grab the bar and have your hand positioned at slightly narrower than shoulder width. Your elbows should be pointed outside. Keeping the bar close to your body lift it till it is at the middle of your chest. Be sure to always have your elbows pointed out throughout the exercise and they should be above the bar at peak contraction.

You don't need to lift it all the way till the bar is at your chin. The reason for this is because some of the emphasis will shift to rotor cuff rotation. Again, you don't want to put too much burden on your rotor cuffs, because they are very easy to injure.

Barbell Upright Rows

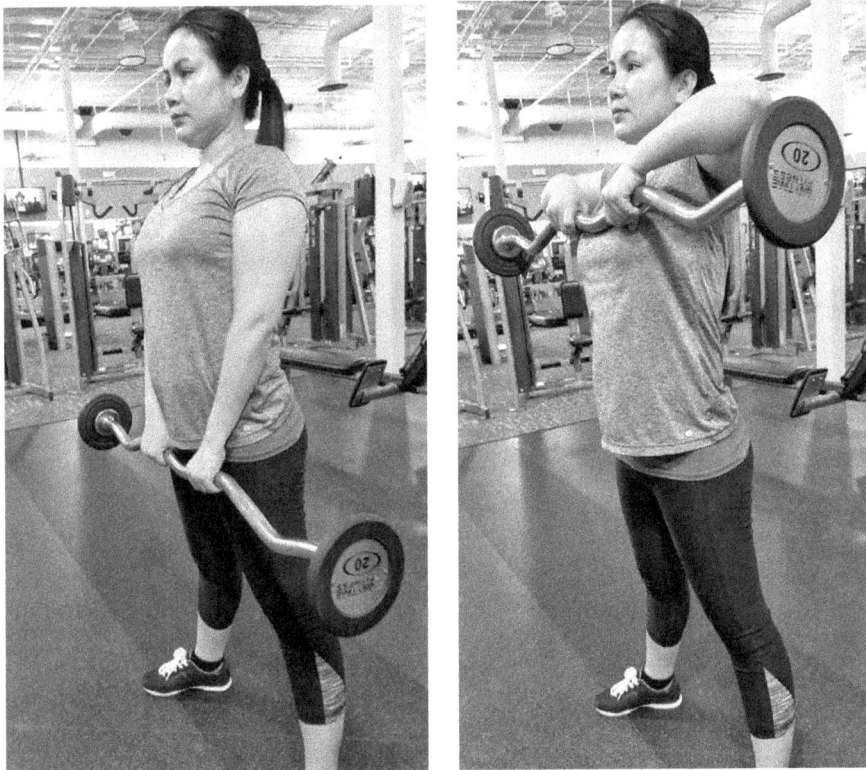

Shiela Garcia

Capable Upright Rows

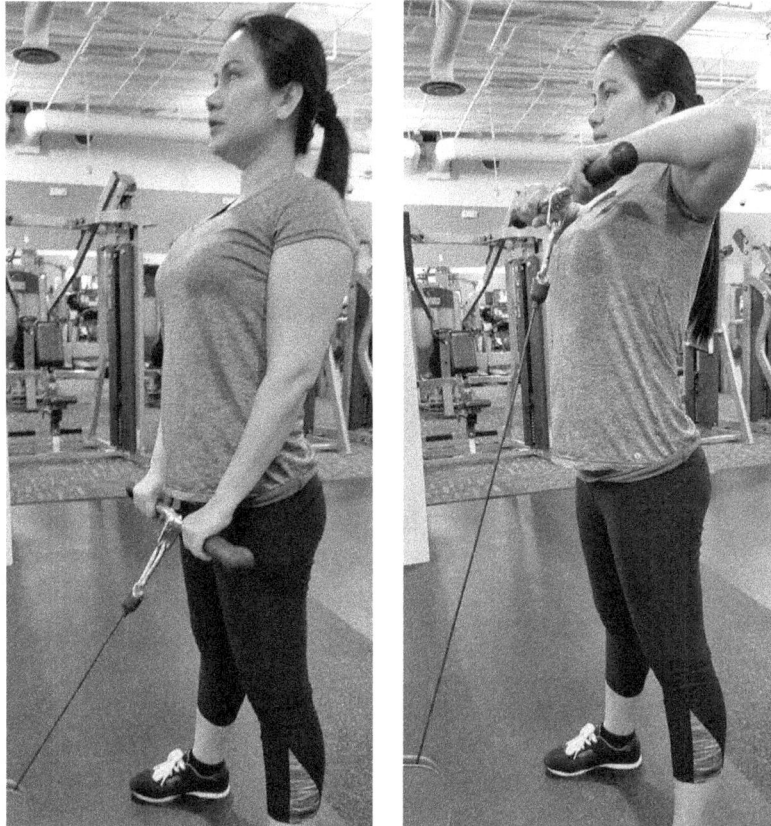

Shiela Garcia

Dumbbell Lateral Flys

You can either do this exercise standing up or sitting down. As always, arch your

back, bend your knees slightly (if you're standing up), and bend your elbows slightly.

Lift your arms up to the sides and be sure that it doesn't go much higher than your

shoulders. The position of your arms at point should be parallel to the floor. If the angle

or position of the dumbbells is slightly tilted then it is still alright, but never have them

perpendicular to the floor.

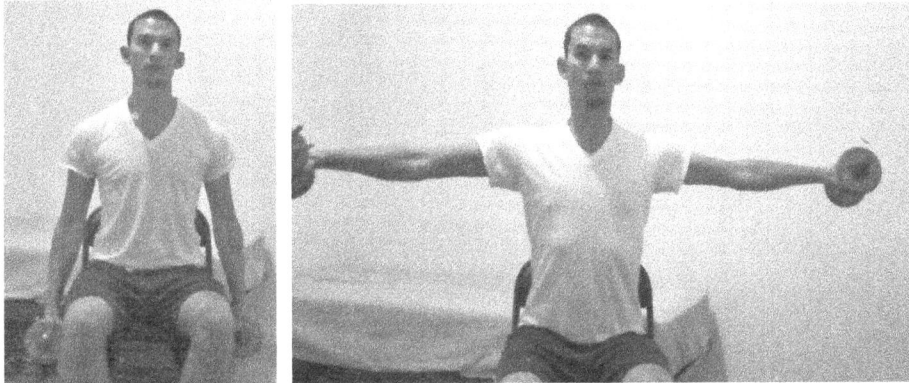

Jaime Augusto Barrientos Jr.

Dumbbell Posterior Flys

This one may be difficult to do for people who have a pre-existing lower back problem. If this is a case for you then you should perform this exercise with light weights while sitting down at the edge of the bench bent down. But if not then this should be performed bent down standing up in order to effectively hit the rear of your deltoids.

With dumbbells in your hands be sure to arch your back. Bend your knees slightly and bend forward till your body is somewhat parallel to the floor. Raise your head up in order to minimize the increase blood pressure going to your head. Your elbows should be slightly bend and pointing out and pointing up as you move. Lift it as high as you can and pause for a second or two at peak contraction.

Be sure the dumbbells you are using are light so you can get a feel for the exercise and for your muscles. You'll see that this exercise not only works out the rear deltoid, but also your back muscles and your rhomboid (located at the center of your back).

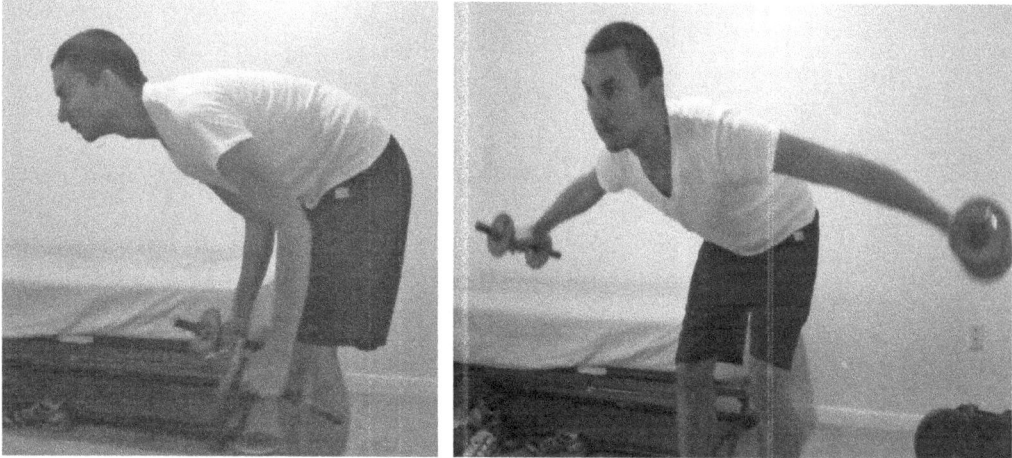

Jaime Augusto Barrientos Jr.

Dumbbell Anterior Flys

Grab a couple of dumbbells. Have them in front of your thighs. Arch your back and bend your elbows slightly. You can either lift the dumbbells together in front of you or you can do it one arm at a time. Which ever way you lift it just make sure the dumbbells are slightly above your shoulders.

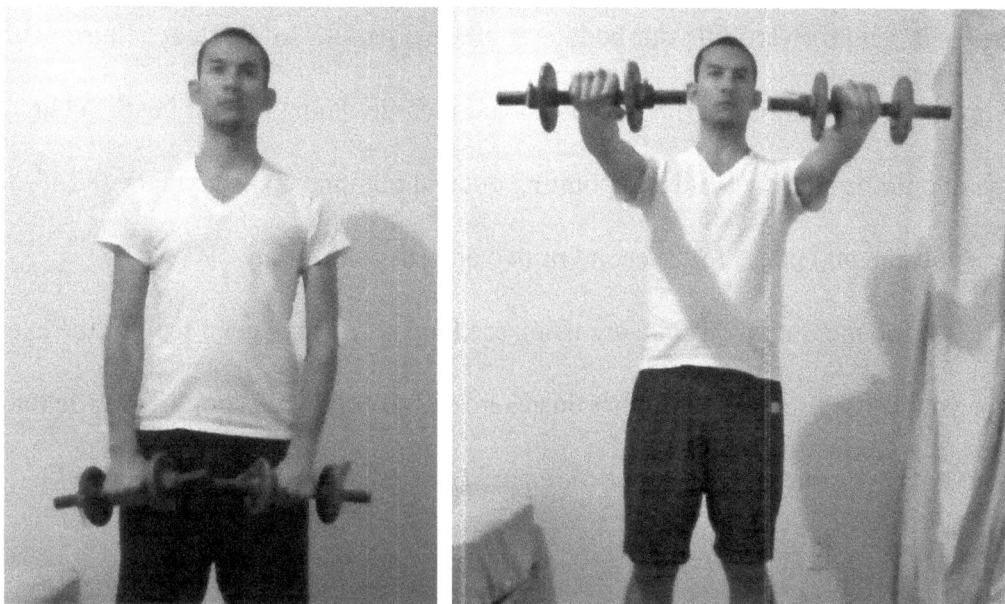

Jaime Augusto Barrientos Jr.

Triceps

These muscles are located at the back of your upper arms between the shoulders and elbows. Triceps are often involved with some of the chest and shoulder exercises such as bench presses and shoulder presses. They can be easily overtrained. I have met trainers in the past who have injured their triceps severely because of it.

Many bodybuilders think that in order to have large upper arms you have to develop your biceps. They tend to forget that the triceps are much larger than the biceps. Why, because triceps consist of three sub-muscles or three heads, while the biceps have two. So if you want to develop large upper arms don't neglect your triceps.

Cable Triceps Extension

This can be done with a short straight bar or with a rope. Stand in front of a pulley machine with a short bar or rope attached to an upper cable. Grab the bar or rope with both hands. Your palms should be facing down if it's the bar. Have your elbows steady at your sides with your arms bent. Be sure your back is arch on this exercise. Now pull the bar down till your arms are straight. It's alright to lock your elbows on this exercise. Be sure to keep your elbows steady throughout the movement.

Short Bar Triceps Extension

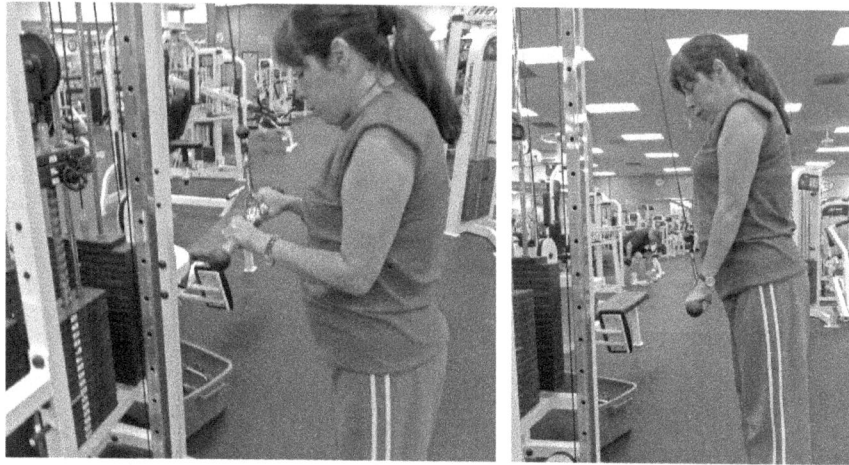

Adriana Garcia

Rope Triceps Extension

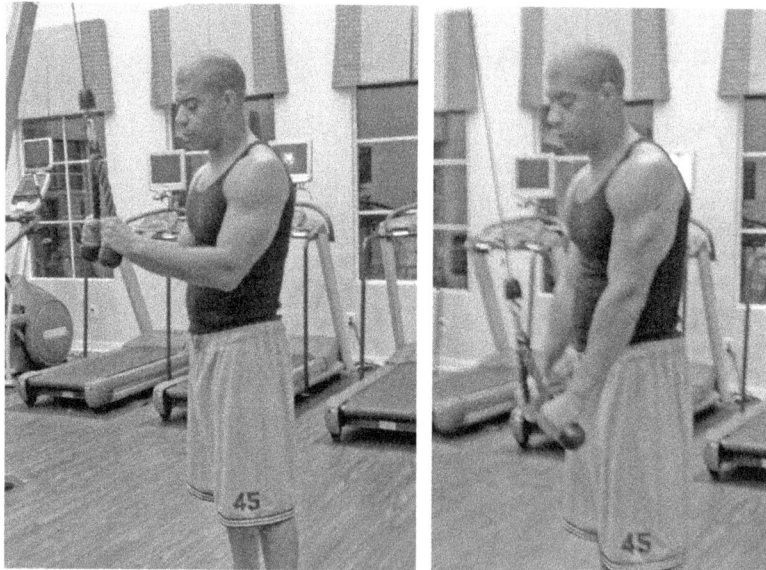

Jarrod Bryant

French Press or Skull Crusher

This particular exercise requires a flat bench and a barbell. You can either use a straight bar or an EZ curling bar. Place the barbell almost at the edge of the bench. Lie flat on your back on the bench. Your head should be below the barbell and your feet should be flat on the floor. Grab the barbell with both hands at shoulder width and raise it up till your arms are straight. This will be your starting point. Lower the barbell till it is behind your head. Just for your safety never lower the barbell in front of your face, because if you do and once you hit positive failure you'll find out why they call it skull crusher. Keep your elbows and upper arms stable throughout the movement.

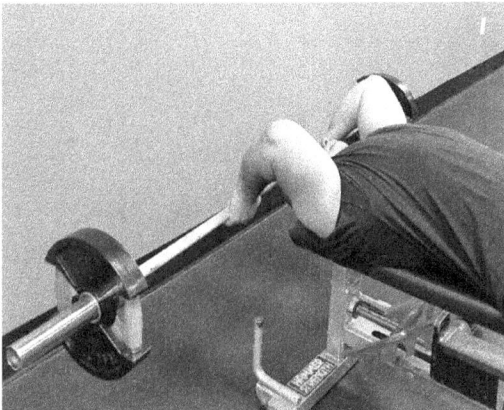

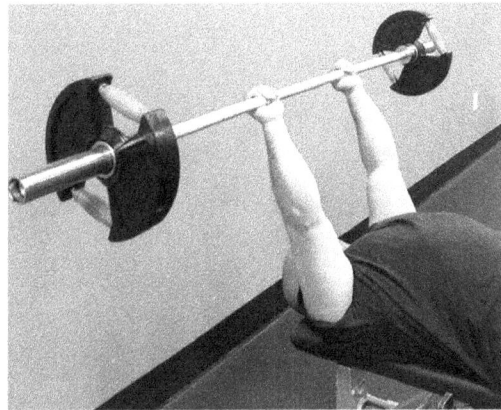

Dumbbell Tricep Extension

You can do this exercise either sitting down or standing up. Grab a dumbbell and raise it up above your head till your arm is straight. This will be your starting point. Slowly lower the dumbbell till it is behind your head. Lift it up till your arm is straight again. Keep your elbow and upper arm stable throughout the movement. Repeat the same procedure to the other arm.

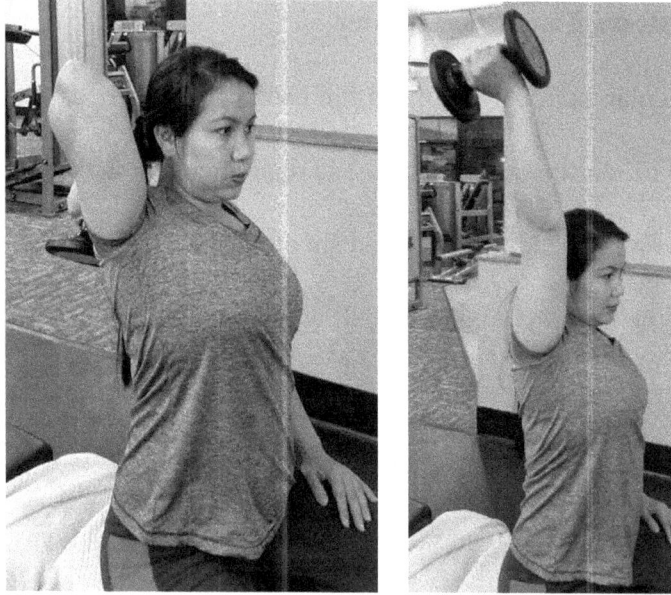

Shiela Garcia

Dips

This exercise requires parallel bars. Your bodyweight will provide the resistance. Place your hands on the parallel bars. Lift yourself up till your arms are straight. This will be your starting point. As you go down be sure to keep your elbows are close to your body. If your elbows are far from your body the emphasis of the exercise will shift primarily to working out your chest. Keep your body straight as you go down and with your head tilted slightly down. This way you keep your balance. Go as far down as you possibly can. Be careful not to get sloppy on your form. The possibility of getting hurt from this exercise is great if you don't pay attention to your form and proper rep scheme.

Some beginners might find this exercise a bit difficult to perform. If it is too difficult then I suggest you skip it for now. You can perform this exercise as soon as you get stronger and better developed.

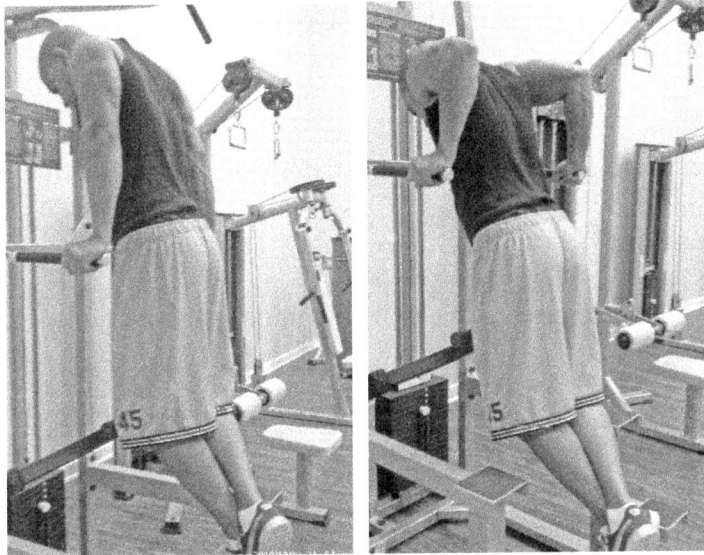

Jarrod Bryant

Biceps

When someone comes up to you and ask, "Let's see your muscles" you don't take off your shirt and show them your chest or back. Neither do you drop your pants down to show them your legs. Rather, you roll up your sleeves and flex your biceps to them. Believe it or not, your biceps serve as an ambassador to your physique. People will often judge how well developed you are according to your biceps.

Well the good news is that biceps do develop rather easily. Just about every person I've trained in the gym has developed their biceps first before any of their body parts. The bad news is that not everyone will develop high peak biceps. Like me, you may end up with well developed biceps that are flat. Indeed, the shape of your biceps is determined by your genes. Of course the same can be said for the rest of your body parts.

Regardless of what your genetics may be, it doesn't mean that you can't develop thick muscular biceps.

Before going into the biceps exercises there's one important thing I need to mention. You must always bend your arms slightly at the extended position when performing any curling exercises. This will help minimize injury to your biceps' tendon.

Barbell Curls

This exercise is performed standing up with your back arched. Grab hold of a barbell with your hands holding it at shoulder width. Bend your elbows slightly while keeping your upper arms and elbows close to your body. Lift the barbell up till your forearms are touching your biceps. Be sure to keep your upper arms stable and do not move your elbows forward.

If a straight barbell hurts your wrist then you should try using the EZ curl bar. The only thing about using an EZ curl bar is that the brachial muscle, which is the muscle that is located between your biceps and triceps, come more into play, but other than that it is quite alright.

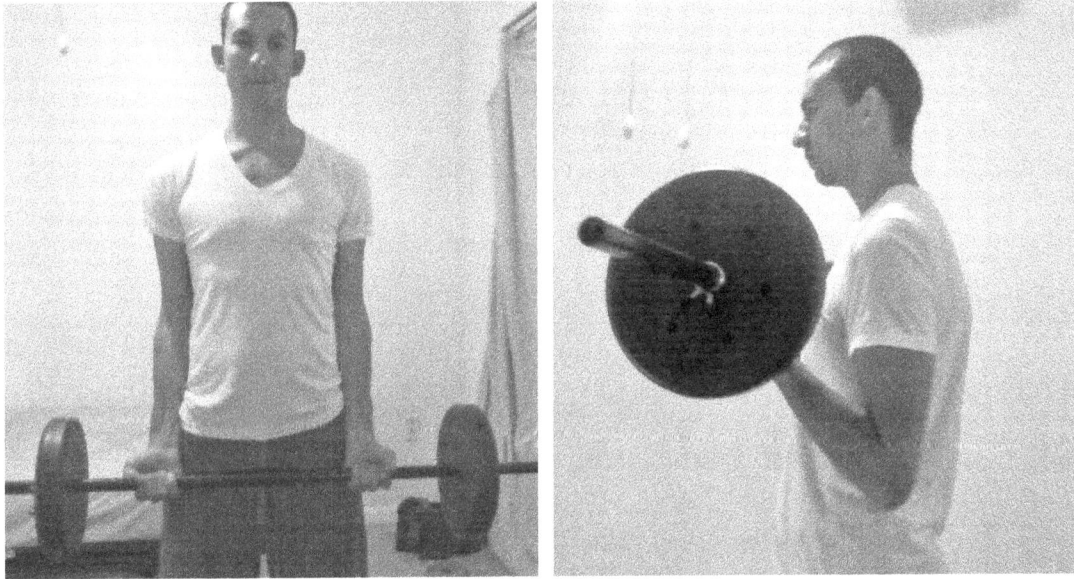

Jaime Augusto Barrientos Jr.

Dumbbell Alternating Curls

Stand straight with your back arched. Grab two dumbbells and have them at your sides. Bend your arms slightly and curl one arm at a time. As you are raising them up for curl be sure to twist the dumbbell at a 90 degree angle. So that when you reach peak contraction the palm of your hand would be facing you.

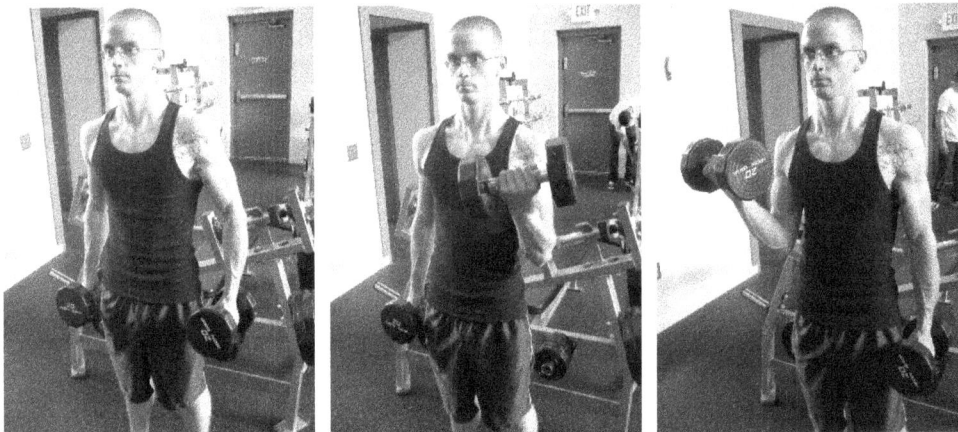

Kyle Babb

Bench Curls

This particular exercise can either be performed by using a barbell, dumbbell, machine, or cable. This is the best exercise you could do for your biceps because it hits them more directly. If you are planning on using a machine to do this then it is even better. Most machines come with a special cam that makes the tension continuous throughout the range of motion. Whereas for barbells and dumbbells the tension minimizes as you get closer to peak contraction and extended position.

When performing this exercise be sure to lean into the arm pad. The top of the arm pad should be up against your arm pits. Bend your arms slightly and perform the exercise. Be sure to take advantage of the continuous tension by holding your peak contraction a second longer than usual.

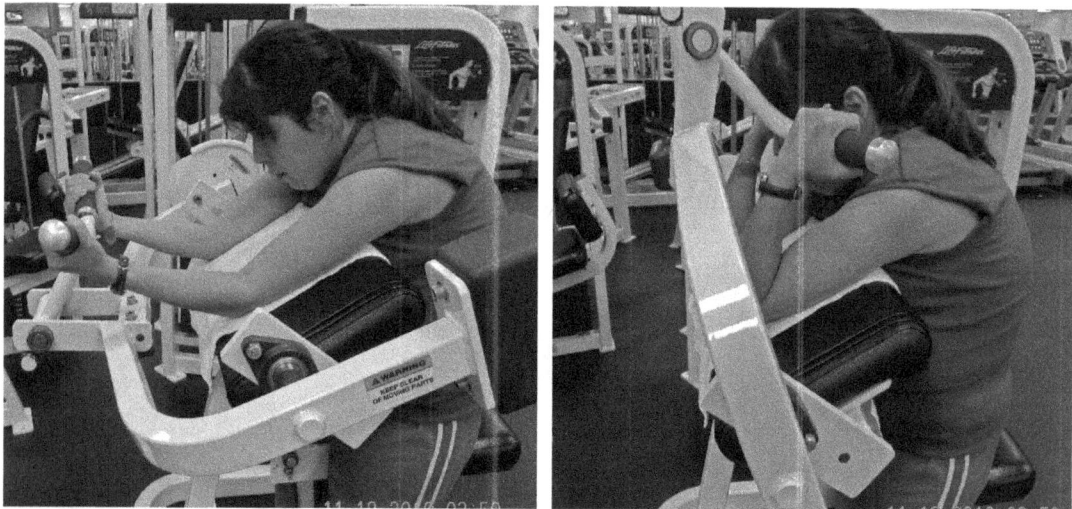

Adriana Garcia

To get the full benefit from this Machine Bench Curls be sure to lean into it.

Forearms

Forearms are one of those muscles that you can do without training. They get a lot of workout just from gripping the weights. They especially get worked out every time you do your biceps and triceps.

Back then I decided to stop working out my forearms due to an injury to my right wrist. It was impossible for me to do wrist curls and reverse wrist curls. I thought for sure that they would shrink or lag behind from the rest of my body parts. I was wrong. My forearms did develop with the rest of my body parts just by gripping hard on the exercises I did. Looking at my log they went from 12 inches to 14 ½ inches and this was from doing no direct forearm training at all.

Now I don't want to say that you should never train your forearms at all. That really is up to you. If you do decide to do them I recommend you incorporate them with your biceps and triceps routine. There are two very direct forearm exercises that I highly recommend: Wrist Curls and Reverse Wrist Curls.

Wrist Curls

You would need to be seated with this particular exercise. Grab a barbell with both hands or with a dumbbell. Place your forearms on your lap and have your wrists extend out from your knees. The palms of your hands should be facing up. Be sure to grip the bar or dumbbell as hard as you can, because part of your forearm development is from the grip itself. Have the barbell or dumbbell go down, which will be your starting point, and then go ahead and curl your wrist.

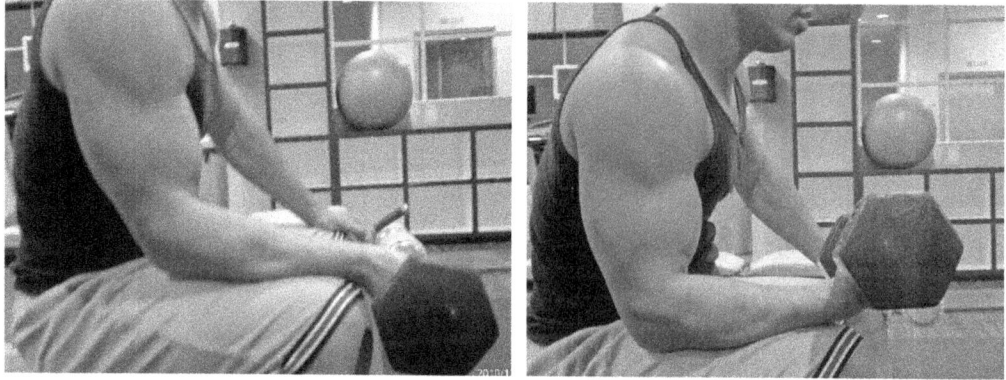

Jarrod Bryant

Reverse Wrist Curls

This exercise is just that, the reverse side of wrist curls. The positioning is very much the same except the palms of your hands are facing down. You do the exact same thing by gripping the bar or dumbbell as hard as you can and then curl your wrist.

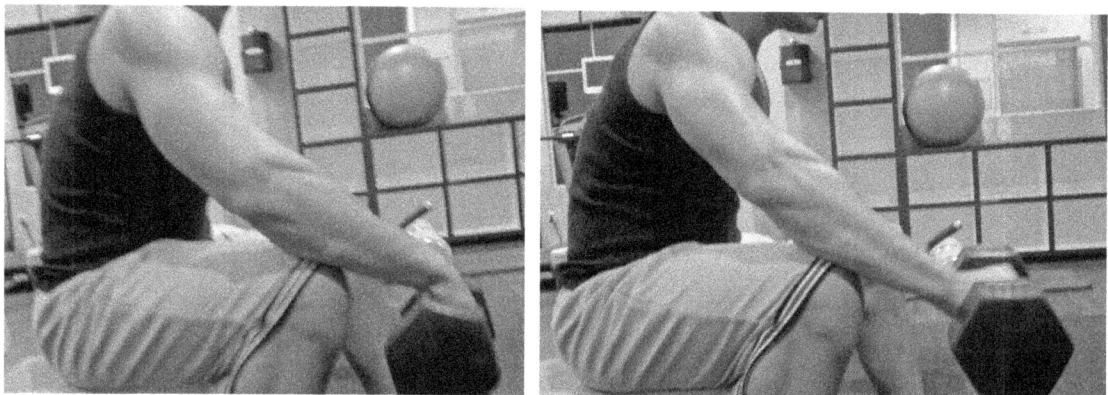

Jarrod Bryant

Abdominals

As biceps seem to be the ambassador for your muscular development, rectus abdominis, abdominals or abs seem to be the ambassador to your fitness level. When people see that you have washboard abs they know that you are fit. Abs are also looked upon as a symbol of health and beauty. Just like those statues from Greece and Rome.

But no matter how well developed your abs may be, if you have layers of fat covering them they will not show. You do have to diet and have a low percentage of body fat in order for them to show. Luckily for you, who happen to be thin, this may not be a problem. The only thing you need to do is develop them.

One of the most common mistakes people make with working out their abs is that they tend to overtrain them. They do a number of reps and sets in the gym thinking that's how it is to develop them. On top of that they tend to do abs every single day. I don't know how people got the notion that ab muscles are different from the rest of the muscles when in truth they are not.

I remember Sergio when he came to workout in my gym. He was a competitive bodybuilder from Mexico and he was preparing for a natural (drugfree) bodybuilding contest that Denny Kakos was promoting in my town, Corona. He already had sharp abs when I first met him. As the contest was getting closer he did abs every single day for almost1 hour before he trained any of his body parts. On the day of the contest he didn't place in the top 10. The sharp abs he had were literally gone. All I saw was a smooth stomach. "What happened?" I remember saying that to my gym buddy when he walked up on stage.

Abdominals are like any muscles in your body. They need to be properly trained. There's no need to do high reps or high sets or to train them more frequently than any of your other muscles. You can train them in the same manner as you train any of your body parts. They will develop the same way. Many bodybuilders think that if you train abs in H.I.T. fashion they would get thicker and they would end up looking like a beer belly. That is simple not true. Abdominals develop better when they are not overtrained.

Many bodybuilders think that there are two parts to abs: upper abs and lower abs. If you look at the medical book of the anatomy chart of the abdominal muscles you'll see that it is just one connection. They are connected to your hips or pelvis and to your ribcage. Just that our belly button gives that illusion that there are two parts to it. So there really is no need to do two separate types of workouts. Just remember the main function of the abs is to stabilize the trunk and to move the body between the ribs and pelvis.

Well what about intercostals and oblique muscles (located at the side of your mid-section)? These are stabilizer muscles as I call them. They are part of the abdominal muscles. They come into play as you workout your abs. So I don't really recommend working them out separately. If you wish to do a direct workout on them you can always do side bends.

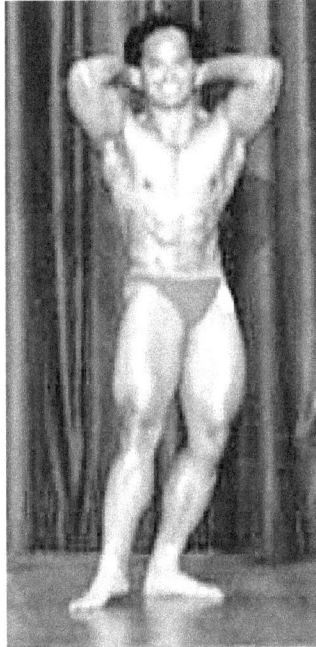

Dumbbell Crunches

Lie flat on the floor and bend your knees. You can either place your feet flat on the floor or on top of a bench. Grab hold of the dumbbell and have it right on top of your chest. Be sure to hold firmly to the dumbbell and make sure that it is manageable. Do your reps by raising your shoulder blades off the floor. Perform this exercise in the same manner as you perform the other exercises.

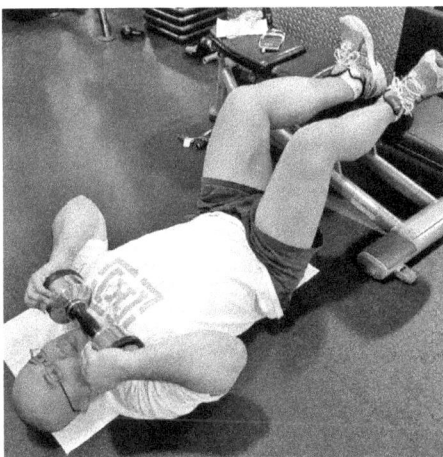

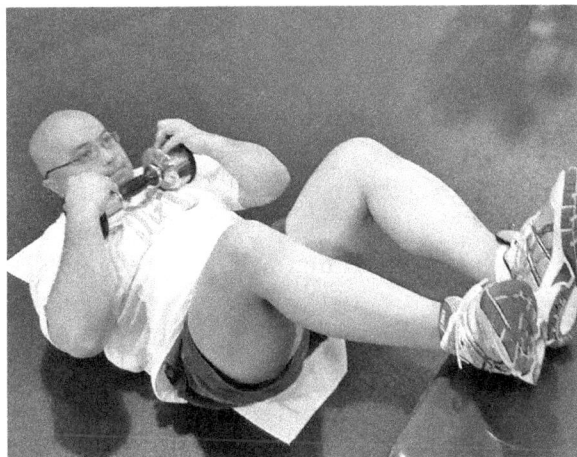

Dumbbell Leg Raises

Lie flat on the floor with your head up and your shoulders off the floor. Place your hands underneath your buttocks. Bend your legs slightly at the knees with your lower back touching the floor. Grab hold of the dumbbell (be sure it's light) with your feet holding it at the handle bar. Now raise your feet up till it is at a diagonal position from the floor. No need to raise them up till your legs is straight up. That will only take the tension away from your abs. Also, do not let your feet down to touch the floor at the extended position for the same reason. If your lower back tends to arch throughout the movement then the weight you are using is too much. Lower the weight and be sure that your lower back never leaves the floor.

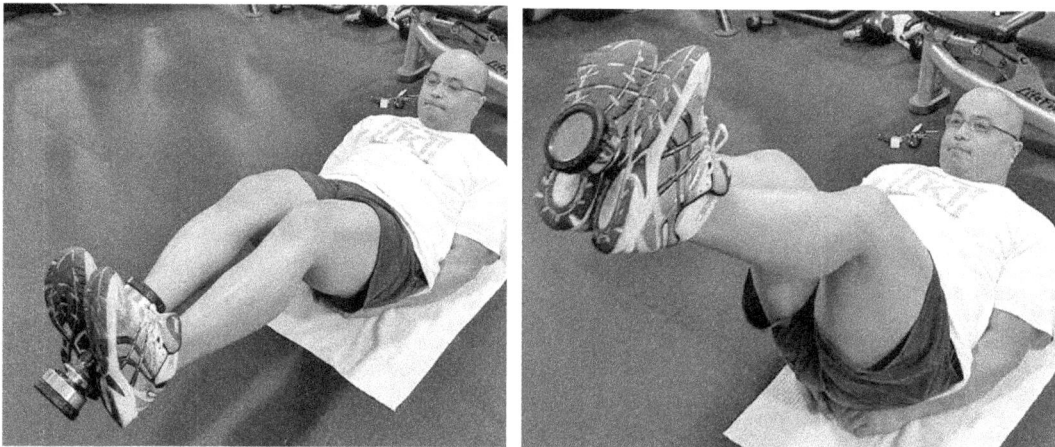

Dumbbell Sit Ups

This exercise may require you to have someone hold your feet or place your feet underneath something that will hold it steady. Bend your legs all the way till your calves and hamstrings are touching together. Grab hold of the dumbbell and place it on your chest. Raise your head and shoulders off the floor as you start the lift. Then raise you whole upper body up till it is close to your legs. Keep your head and shoulders stable

146

throughout the range of motion. Your back should be curve and not arching. Arching your back on this movement will put more emphasis on the solar flexes and this may cause a possible injury. You must keep your back curve throughout the range of motion in order to make this a very effective workout for your abs.

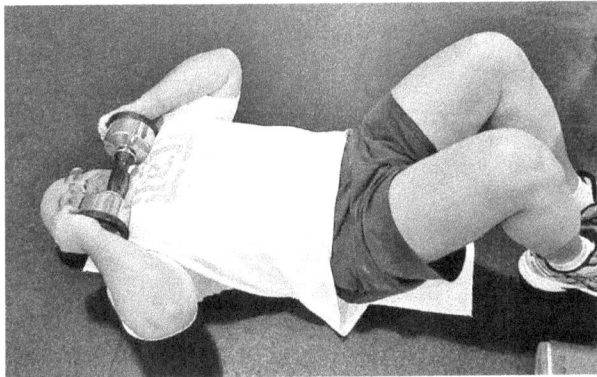

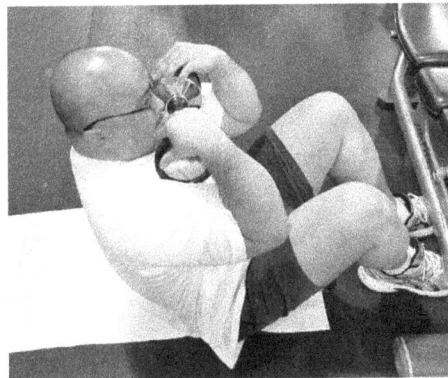

"One of the greatest experiences in life is achieving personal goals that others said would be, 'Impossible to attain.' Be proud of your success and share your story with others."

--Robert Cheeke

PART V

The Importance of Warming Up

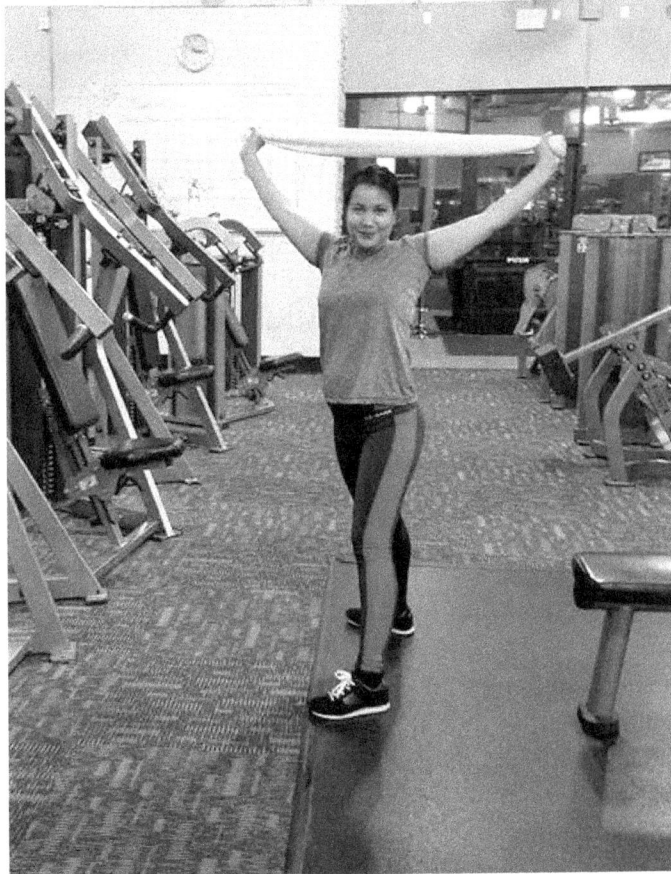

Shiela Garcia doing her warm ups before the workout.

CHAPTER 21

WARM UPS

I received an email once from a guy in England who claimed to have never done any sort of warm ups before his workouts. In his email he told me his motivation was his warm ups. He then explained to me how wrong he was. He mentioned how he loaded his barbell for his bench press at 315lbs. On his first rep when he was doing the positive lift he felt his right pectoral muscles ripping from the inside. He barely got the weight up and back on the rack. Normally he could do 6 reps with the weight, but on that day he barely made one.

He went home that same day without continuing his chest workout or any workout for that matter. He treated his injury by alternating between the hot pad and cold pack of ice and he asked me if this was right. I immediately emailed him back and told him to go see a doctor right away and have an MRI done. A couple of days later he emailed me back and thanked me. According to his doctor who reviewed his MRI that he had a partial tear on his right pectoral. He recommended microscopic surgery to repair it. I truly believe that this could have been avoided if he would have done some proper warm up before engaging on a heavy set of bench press.

It doesn't matter what physical activity you are planning to engage in, whether be in weight training, speed walking, jogging, swimming, playing tennis, or even golf you must always perform warm up first. Warming up not only helps your muscles prepare for the physical activity it also helps prepare you mentally for it.

During the warm ups you should visualize how you are going to do your workouts and psych yourself up for it. During my stretching warm ups I visualize my workouts. In my mind's eye I'm performing the exercises already. I saw myself doing more reps and weights. Before I even engage myself in a workout in my mind I've already done them.

During my warm ups where I am lifting light weights I visualize my muscles developing and getting stronger. I psych myself up in reaching and surpassing my target rep before I train that particular body part. So as you can see I am extremely motivated, I'm in the zone sort of speaking. I am so extremely focus that my surroundings no longer concern me.

It is important that you get in to this type of mentality or zone. It is the best way to get a productive workout. So warming up is not just about getting the blood flow going, your heart slightly elevated, or your body temperature to rise up, but it's also about visualization and psyching yourself up for the actual H.I.T. workout.

Stretching

There has been a debate among fitness gurus as to whether or not stretching is a form of physical exercise. Well if we look at what physical exercise does for you we can see that it burns calories, helps you increase strength and mass, improve your cardiovascular system, and increase your basal metabolic rate. So is stretching a form of physical exercise? The answer to that in my book is no, but it does improve your flexibility and it somewhat improve the blood flow.

Stretching does feel good though. If you've been driving for 6 to 8 hours or been working in front of a computer all day or studying for an important test you know that your body tends to tense up due to stress. Stretching helps alleviate such tension. For me going to a gym after an 8 hour work day and a 2 hour drive from a freeway, stretching before my workout helps me relax and loosen up.

The goal with stretching is not to see how far you can stretch your muscles and tendons. You only run the risk of actually injuring them since they are in such a compromised position. Your goal is also not to try and increase your flexibility. You can do this by performing your exercises in a full range of motion. Your goal is to stretch in a comfortable position in order to loosen up the muscles and tendons and to also get yourself in the zone.

When stretching be sure that you feel the individual muscles being stretched. Hold that stretched position for 10 to 15 or even 20 seconds before moving on to the next muscle. Only stretch the muscles that you are going to workout. But if you think you would feel better by doing a total body stretch then by all means, do it.

I highly recommend that when you are in a stretched position that you don't bounce around. This can lead to a potential injury. Your stretches should be a nice and steady hold.

I don't recommend that you do stretching during your workout. It would just be pointless to stretch the muscle that has already been stretched during the workout. Like I said before, they were stretched during full range of motion.

Calves

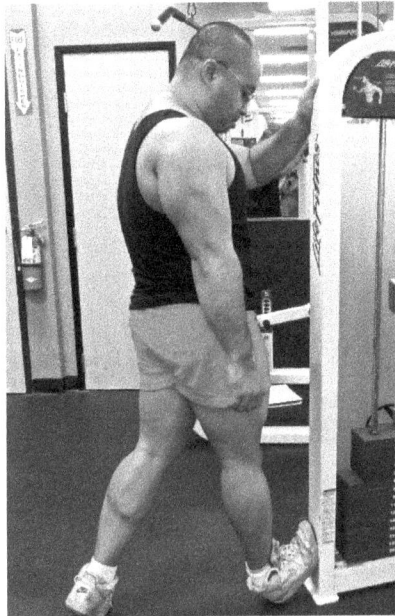

Be sure to lock your knee during the stretch.

Thighs

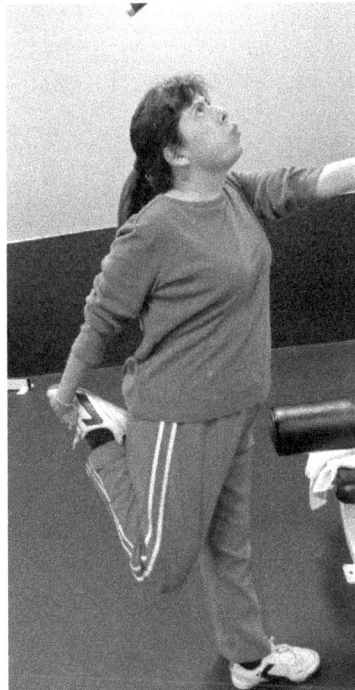

Adriana Garcia

Hamstrings

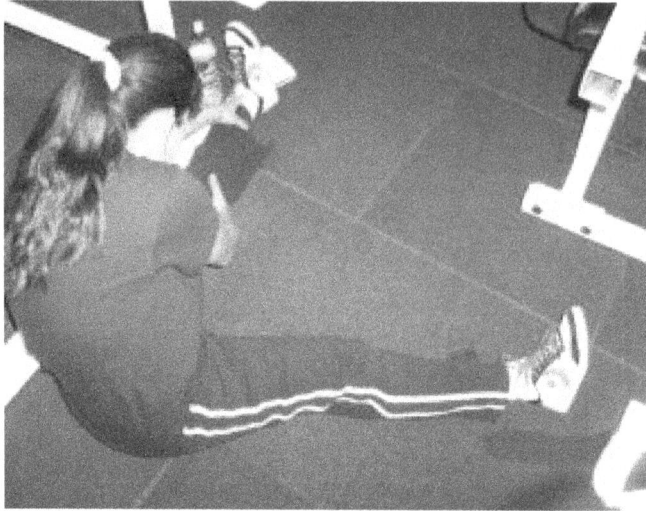

Adriana Garcia

When you do this make sure your legs are straight with knees lock.

Chest

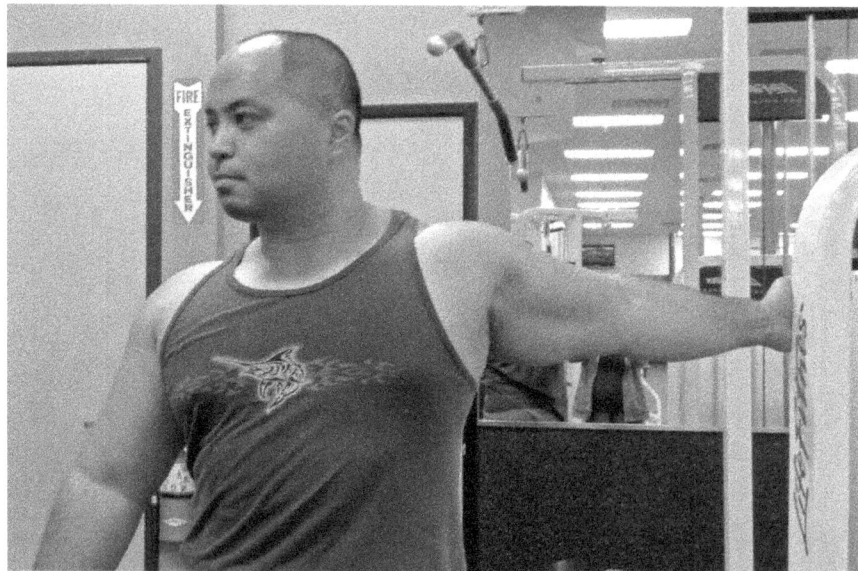

Back

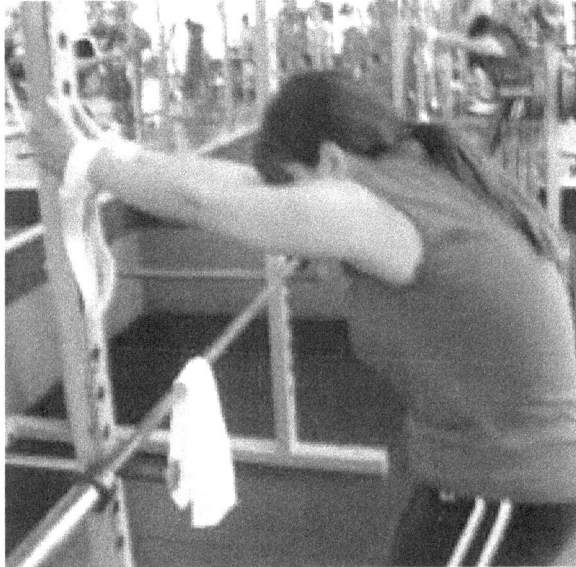

Adriana Garcia

Your arms have to be relaxed as you stretch your back.

Lower Back

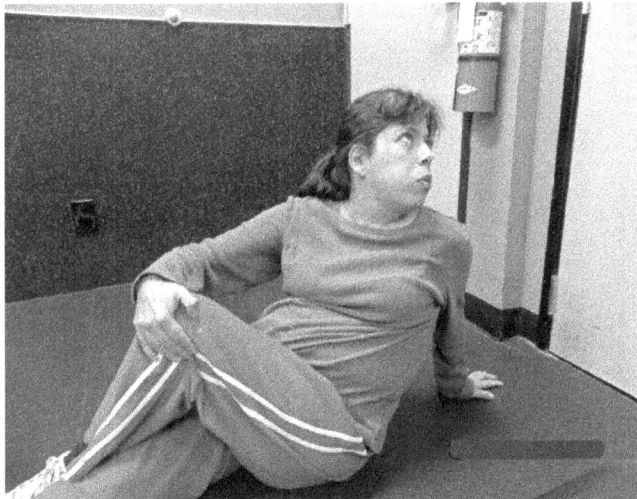

Adriana Garcia

One leg over the other and twist a quarter of a way. If you hear your back pop it's quite alright, but don't overdo it.

Toe Raises

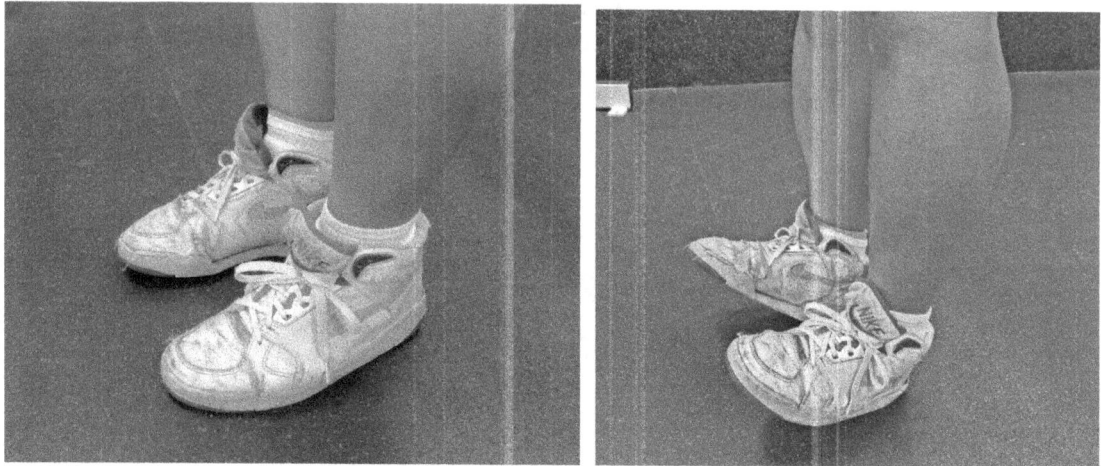

Not really a stretch, but this is to avoid shin splits during calf raises. Make this as part of your warm ups. This works out your tibialis anterior which will help balance things out with your calves. Do 30 to 50 of these toe raises. Runners will benefit from this as well.

Shoulders

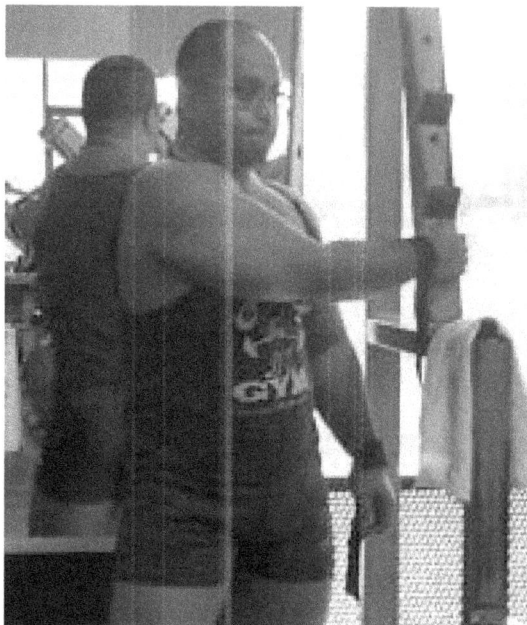

Make sure your arm is completely relax during the stretch

Triceps

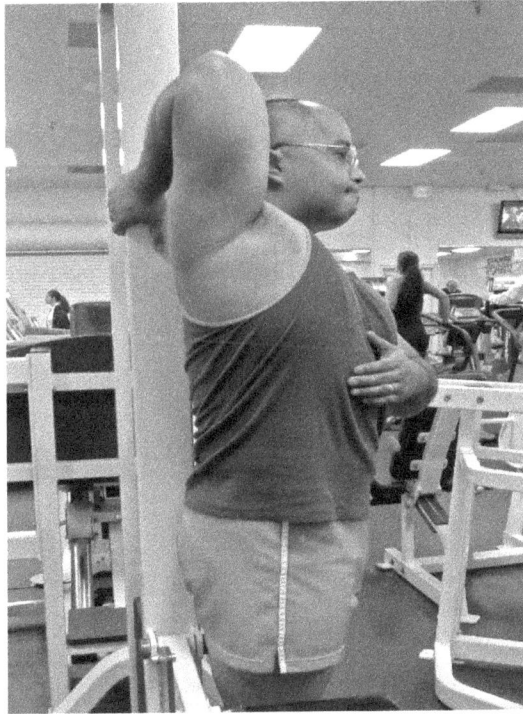

Biceps

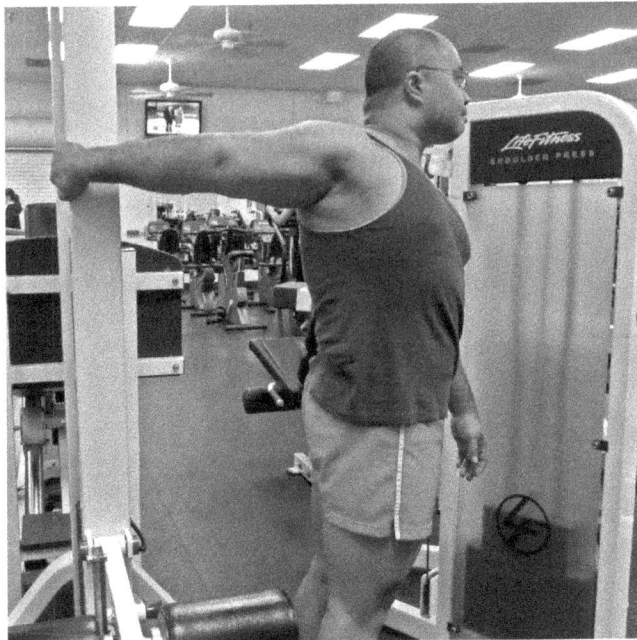

Forearms

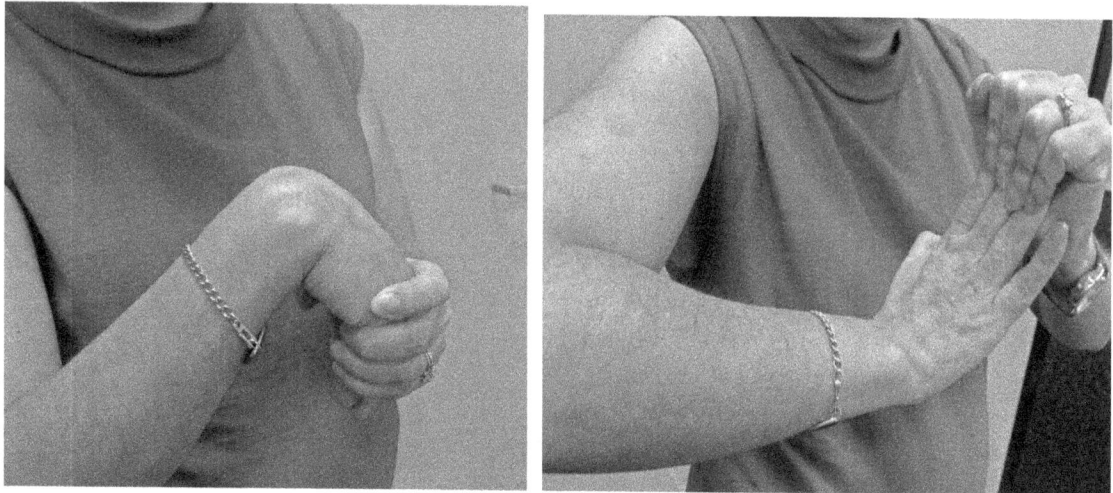

Adriana Garcia

Abs, Chest, and Ribcage Stretch

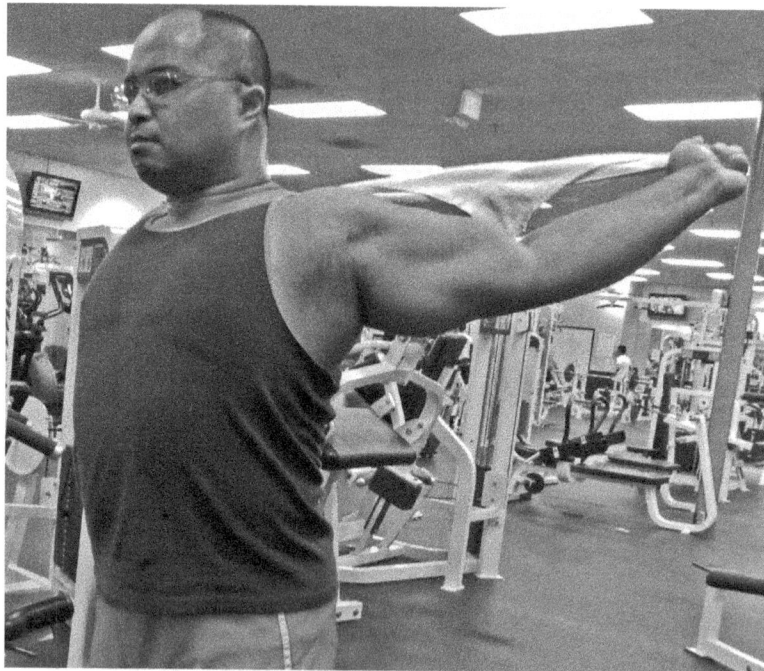

Light Weight Warm Ups

Once you are done with stretching go ahead and do light weight warm ups for that particular exercise that you are planning on doing. The goal here is to prepare the muscles for the hard workouts by increasing the blood flow to those particular muscles and to elevate your body temperature and your heart rate slightly. This will also help minimize injury.

So for example if you are doing chest and you plan on doing bench press first and then dumbbell flys then you do your warm ups with the bench press. If your maximum bench press is at 225lbs then I suggest you start your warm ups with 95lbs and do 15 reps. Rest briefly once done and add weights to the bar and do your second warm up with 135lbs for 10 reps. By now your chest muscle should feel warmed up. Go ahead and do your 225lbs bench press. Once you are done with your bench press you can go ahead and do dumbbell flys. There's no need to do warm ups with dumbbell flys because your chest should still be hot from the bench press you just did.

If you are doing a total body workout then I suggest you do your warm ups by doing the whole body. It wouldn't matter which exercises you choose to do as long as you do high reps with it at about 15 to 20. Since the weights you use are light then there's no need to rest in-between warm ups. As soon as you finish with one warm up exercise go ahead and jump on the next one as quickly as you can till you get your whole body parts warmed up. This will slightly increase the rate of your cardio and the temperature of your body.

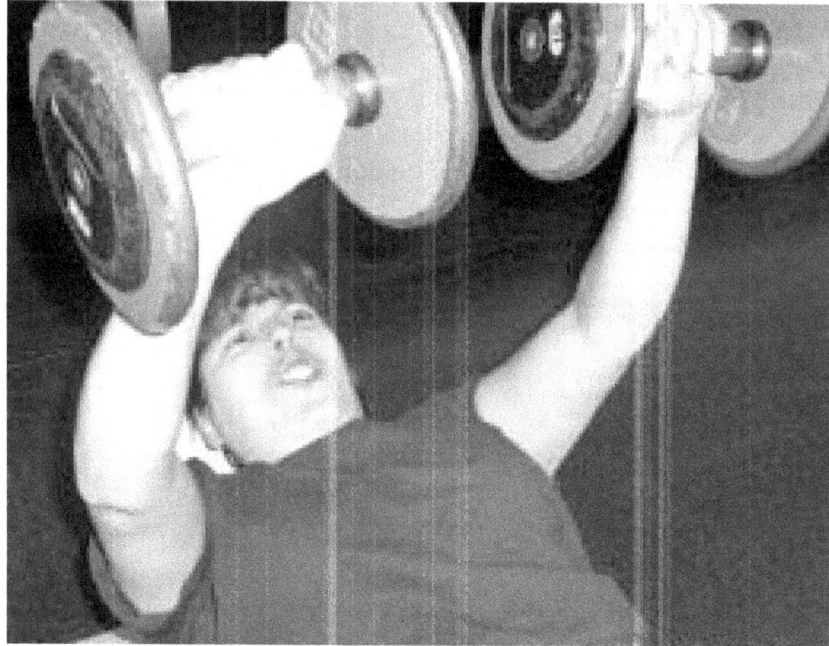

Adriana Garcia

Warm Ups are not workouts

Be careful not to turn your warm ups into workouts. Doing too many warm ups can turn into a workout that can lead to overtraining. Meaning if your warm ups is causing your muscles to fatigue before your actual workout then this can cause overtraining. Not only that, but too many warm ups can actual affect your workout performance.

There's no need to do pyramids where you do 5 sets or more. This is normally done by increasing the weights you use while decreasing your reps. The first 3 sets or so of this are considered warm ups, while the last 2 sets or so are the actual workouts. This particular type of set sequence is very popular in the gym. But it can only lead to overtraining, which is something you must avoid.

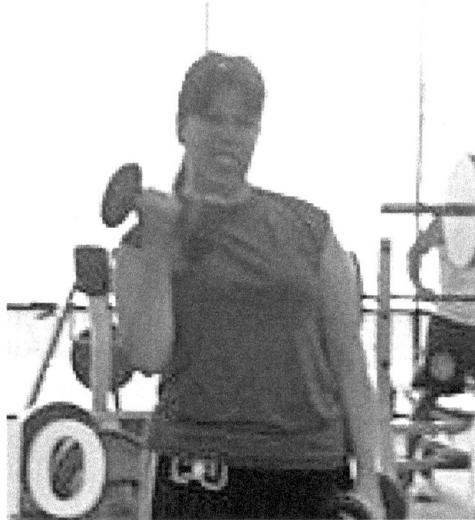

Adriana Garcia

Be careful not to turn your warm ups into workouts.

Cooling Down

Once you are done with your workout you would be at an elevated aerobic state. Meaning your breathing and your heart rate is at a rapid pace. This is normal and it may take you 10 minutes or so to have your aerobic state back to normal. It's not a good idea to just go and exit the gym immediately without cooling down from it first.

During that time I recommend you stay standing and drink some water. I don't recommend you sit down or lie down. By sitting you may have the tendency to slouch with your head down. This can hamper your breathing. Lying down may make you feel dizzy or light headed and you may find yourself trying to recover from that as well. You breathe better when you are standing up with your head straight or slightly tilted back. It's alright if you want to lean or hold on to something, but be sure your body is straight.

There's no need to do stretches after your workout. The muscles and tendons are at their weakest state and to top it off there's an increase amount of blood in them, which may give you the feeling of being pumped. I recall back then how my training partner and I used to jog for 3 miles a day. After our run my training partner's thighs would feel very tight and pumped from the run. One day he decided to stretch them and I clearly recall how he ended up straining or pulling something from his left thigh. At the time he didn't know that he injured it till the next day when he had problems walking with his left leg. It took him almost a week or so to fully recover. So to stretch them at this state is not advisable.

PART VI

Total Body Workout

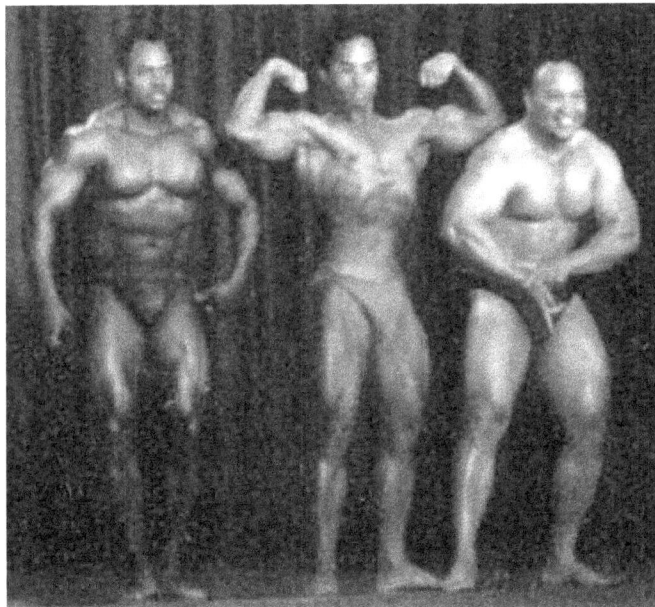

Me at the middle

CHAPTER 22

TOTAL BODY WORKOUT

Phase I

When I first learned about total body workout from Dr. Ellington Darden's books I was first skeptical about it. I was so used to doing 20 sets for large muscles and 10-12 sets for smaller ones. When I did finally came around and tried it I couldn't believe how much progress I made from it. I added 20lbs of muscle mass in a short period of time. And I was only doing 1 set of exercise per body part! My friends from the gym thought I was taking steroids because of the quick gains. My clients who I put through the same workout routine experienced the same thing.

Total body workout is very effective because it is systematic. Our body works in a systematic way because of our recovery ability. That means all of the muscles that got worked out would all need to recover together before the next total body workout.

Whereas in a split body workout, you workout a couple of body parts at a time and you allocate time for them to recover before your next workout for different body parts. It doesn't take advantage of the systematic way of recovery like what the total body workout does. But split body workout is indeed necessary later on in your training, which I will explain later.

I've found that total body workout to be very effective for beginners. To those of you who have never done any sort of training this is the best place to start. To those of you who have worked out before and never been able to get rid of their skinny self I recommend you start here as well.

Total Body Routine

Phase I

This routine is set up so that you do a mixture of compound and isolation exercises for different body parts. It is also set up in a cycle where you start off with legs first and then upper body one week and then the next week you do upper body first and then legs and so forth. This way different body parts get worked out first. Why, because your energy level is usually at its highest at the very beginning of the workout and diminishes as you progress within the workout.

Be sure not to turn your workout routine into a high level aerobic routine. There are many H.I.T. advocates out there that prefer you move from one exercise to another as fast as possible with little to no rest in-between exercises, even when your heart rate and your breathing is at its peak. The problem with this is that your muscles are oxygen depraved and your cardiovascular compromises your muscles full capability.

Rest if you need too in order to lower your aerobic rate before moving to the next exercise. This way your muscles are not starving for oxygen. Don't rest too long though where your body starts to cool off. With time and experience you'll get better at it and your rest period between exercises would become less.

Perform one set per exercise to positive failure. Set your target rep at 8. Be sure to do total body stretches and total body warm ups before engaging your H.I.T. workout routine. Be sure to do proper rep scheme that I described on Chapter 17.

Do your workout twice a week. You can choose which days of the week you want to perform them as long as you get 2 to 3 days rest in-between. Below are the type of exercises I recommend, but you can choose or substitute the type of exercises you wish to use.

Week 1

Monday	Thursday
Standing Calf Raises	Seated Calf Raises
Leg Press	Leg Extensions
Leg Curls	Leg Curls
Bench Press	Incline Dumbbell Flys
Wide Pulldowns	Cable Pullovers
Upright Rows	Dumbbell Lateral Flys
Dips	Cable Triceps Extension
Barbell Curls	Machine Bench Curls
Dumbbell Crunches	Dumbbell Leg Raises

Week 2

Monday	Thursday
Incline Bench Press	Pec Deck
Seated Rows	Dumbbell Rows
Military Press	Barbell Upright Rows
Dumbbell Triceps Extension	French Press
Alternating Dumbbell Curls	Barbell Curls
Squats	Leg Press
Leg Curls	Leg Curls
Seated Calf Raises	Standing Calf Raises
Dumbbell Sit Ups	Dumbbell Leg Raises

Week 3

Monday	Thursday
Dumbbell Leg Raises	Dumbbell Sit Ups
Dips	Dumbbell Overhead Extension
Bench Curl	Dumbbell Alternating Curls
Standing Calf Raises	Seated Calf Raises
Leg Extension	Squats
Leg Curls	Leg Curls
Machine Bench Press	Cable Crossovers
Machine Rows	Wide Pulldowns
Cable Upright Rows	Machine Military Press

Repeat the Cycle

CHAPTER 23

TOTAL BODY WORKOUT
Phase II

As you get stronger and bigger from Total Body Workout Phase I you will soon find that you are overtraining from it. This means that you are no longer generating progress anymore by ways of strength or muscular gain. This is known as a *plateau*. If you find yourself in this predicament don't be quick to jump ahead and do phase II. There are certain things you must analyze first before making this move.

The first thing you need to analyze is your nutritional intake. Are you getting sufficient amount of calories to supply the needs of your developed muscles? Remember, muscles that you have gained from your workout will require a bit more calories than before because of their energy output and plus bigger muscles need more calories to begin with. If you decided to up your calories, be sure to do it where your nutrients remain in balance: 60% Carbohydrate, 30% Protein, and 10% Fat.

The second thing you need to analyze is your rest. Are you getting sufficient amount of sleep? This means are you giving yourself 8 hours or more of sleep a day that your body requires. Lack of sleep can deeply affect your progress in two ways. First it robs you of the energy your muscles need during the day in order to generate an effective workout. Second it robs you of recuperative ability in order for your muscles to generate progress.

The third thing you must analyze is your stress level. Are there certain things in your life that is giving you high stress level? Stress is indeed a part of our lives. We all have it, but unfortunately some have it more than others. High level of stress usually leads to release of certain hormones that are responsible for our fight or flight response. It can rob you of your energy level and it can affect you both physically and psychologically.

I've experienced high stress level in my life where it has caused me to lose 20lbs of my muscles and affected my bowel movement causing me to develop a symptom known as IBS (Irritable Bowel Syndrome). If you are experiencing high level of stress in your life I recommend that you see your doctor right away.

Alright, if you have analyzed all these and they all checked out OK and you honestly haven't made any progress at all for the past couple of months then you are ready to move on to the next phase. Phase II cuts your workout down to almost a half. You will be spending less time in the gym by doing fewer exercises. This means that you'll have more energy to get through your workout and more energy to recuperate better.

Total Body Routine

Phase II

At this phase the exercises are more spread out. You won't be doing your thighs along with your hamstrings or your back along with your chest or biceps along with your triceps. But you will do a combination of exercises that belongs to different muscle groups throughout your workouts.

Perform one set per exercise to positive failure. Set your target rep at 8. Do the proper rep scheme that I described on Chapter 17. Stretch only the body parts you plan to workout on and do the same for warm ups as well. Below are the exercises I recommend, you can choose or substitute the type of exercises you wish to use.

Week 1

Monday	*Thursday*
Squats	Leg Curls
Bench Press	Wide Pulldowns
Upright Rows	Posterior Flys
Dips	Barbell Curls
Dumbbell Sit Ups	Wrist Curls

Week 2

Monday	**Thursday**
Dumbbell Flys	Leg Press
Military Press	Seated Rows
Triceps Extension	Dumbbells Lateral Flys
Seated Calf Raises	Barbell Curls
Hanging Leg Raises	Reverse Wrist Curls

Week 3

Monday	**Thursday**
Upright Rows	Military Press
Incline Bench Press	Dumbbell Rows
Leg Curls	Leg Extension
French Press	Alternating Dumbbell Curls
Dumbbell Crunches	Wrist Curls

Repeat the Cycle

PART VII

Split Body Workout

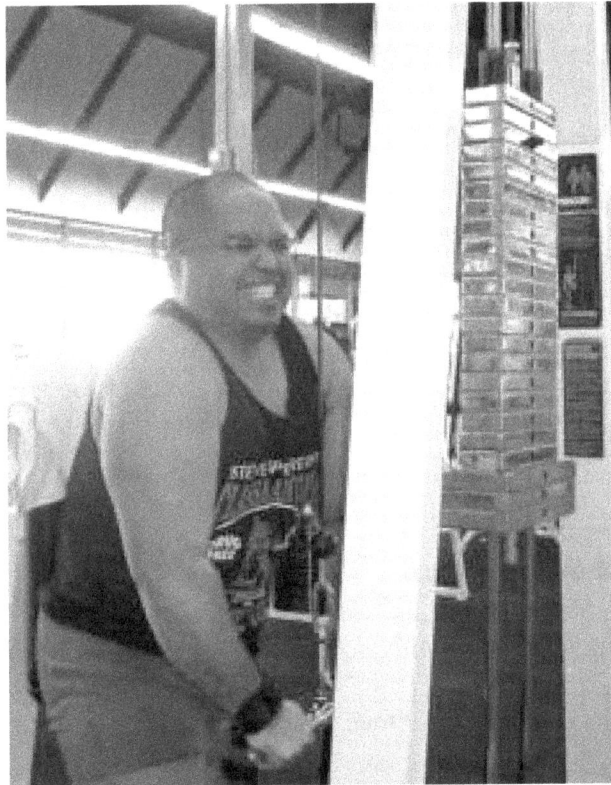

CHAPTER 24

SPLIT BODY WORKOUT

As effective total body workout may be, eventually you would have to come to this phase, split body workout. For me, back then, I had to split my workout routine because I have gotten strong from doing my exercises. I remember how I could do 355lbs of squats and by the time I was done with it I felt like I didn't have much energy left to devout to rest of the exercises. It was the same thing too for my back and chest. Large muscle groups, especially legs, will take a lot out of you. When you hit a plateau and you start to feel drained after your workout then it is time to move on to split body workout.

In the split body workout you would have to combine both compound exercises and isolation exercises for your major muscle groups such as the thigh, back, and chest. Shoulder muscles, triceps and biceps come into play when back and chest muscles are being worked out. So for the sake of doing less workout in order to improve your recovery ability and your energy level you would do them separately.

Stretching and Warm Ups

With stretching you should only stretch the body parts you plan on working out. The same thing goes for your warm ups. Once your muscles are relaxed from the stretching go ahead and begin with the warm ups. Instead of doing the entire warm ups before the workouts the warms ups will be done from within the workout.

With the warm ups I prefer you only do 2 sets of 15 and 10 reps from it. The purpose of the warm up is to prepare the muscles for the heavy set workout. Be sure it is light where you can do 15 reps easily. Increase the weight slightly and do 10 reps easily.

Below are some of the samples you can do for your split body routine. I put it in different options according to the different functions of the muscles. You can choose from it if you wish or you can mix them up and do them in different sequence. The asterisk (*) that you see next to the exercise is where you are going to perform your 2 warm up sets. Again, be sure to do proper form and proper rep scheme that I described on Chapter 17. Always train to positive failure:

Option A

Opposing Muscle Groups

Week 1

Monday	Thursday
<u>Chest</u>	<u>Shoulders</u>
Machine Bench Press*	Barbell Upright Rows*
Dumbbell Flys	Posterior Dumbbell Flys
	Anterior Dumbbell Flys
<u>Back</u>	
Wide Pulldowns*	<u>Abs</u>
Dumbbell Rows	Slow Dumbbell Sit Ups*

Week 2

Monday	Thursday
<u>Triceps</u>	<u>Thighs</u>
Cable Triceps Extension*	Leg Press*
	Leg Extension
<u>Biceps</u>	
Barbell Curls*	<u>Hamstring</u>
	Leg Curls*
<u>Forearms</u>	
Wrist Curls	<u>Calves</u>
Reverse Wrist Curls	Calf Raises*

Repeat the Cycle

Option B

Push/Pull Muscle Groups

Week 1

Monday	Thursday
<u>Chest</u>	<u>Back</u>
Incline Bench Press*	Seated Rows*
Dumbbell Flys	Cable Pullovers
<u>Triceps</u>	<u>Biceps</u>
French Press*	Alternating Dumbbell Curls*
<u>Abs</u>	<u>Forearms</u>
Slow Dumbbell Sit Ups*	Wrist Curls
	Reverse Wrist Curls

Week 2

Monday	Thursday
<u>Shoulders</u>	<u>Thighs</u>
Upright Rows*	Squats*
Military Press*	Leg Extension
Dumbbell Lateral Flys	
Dumbbell Posterior Flys	<u>Hamstring</u>
	Leg Curls*
<u>Abs</u>	
Dumbbell Lying Leg Raises*	<u>Calves</u>
	Calf Raises*

Repeat the Cycle

Option C

Complimentary Muscle Groups

Week 1

Monday	Thursday
Chest	Back
Machine Press*	Wide Pulldowns*
Pec Deck	Dumbbell Rows
Shoulders	Shoulders
Dumbbell Anterior Flys*	Cable Lateral Flys*
	Dumbbell Posterior Flys
Abs	
Dumbbell Leg Raises*	

Week 2

Monday	Thursday
Monday	*Thursday*

Triceps	Thigh
Dips*	Machine Leg Press*
	Leg Extensions
Biceps	
Machine Bench Curls*	Hamstring
	Leg Curls*
Forearms	
Wrist Curls	Calves
Reverse Wrist Curls	Calf Raises*
	Abs
	Dumbbell Sit Ups*

Repeat the Cycle

Whichever option you choose be sure to stick with it for 10 to 12 weeks and then change your exercises around or you can even change your options around. So that this way your body never gets used to doing the same exercises or the same sequence. You can choose whichever exercises you want to perform so long as you have both compound and isolation exercises for major body parts and isolation exercises for minor ones.

"You don't always get what you wish for. You get what you work for."

--Anonymous

PART VIII

Questions and Answers

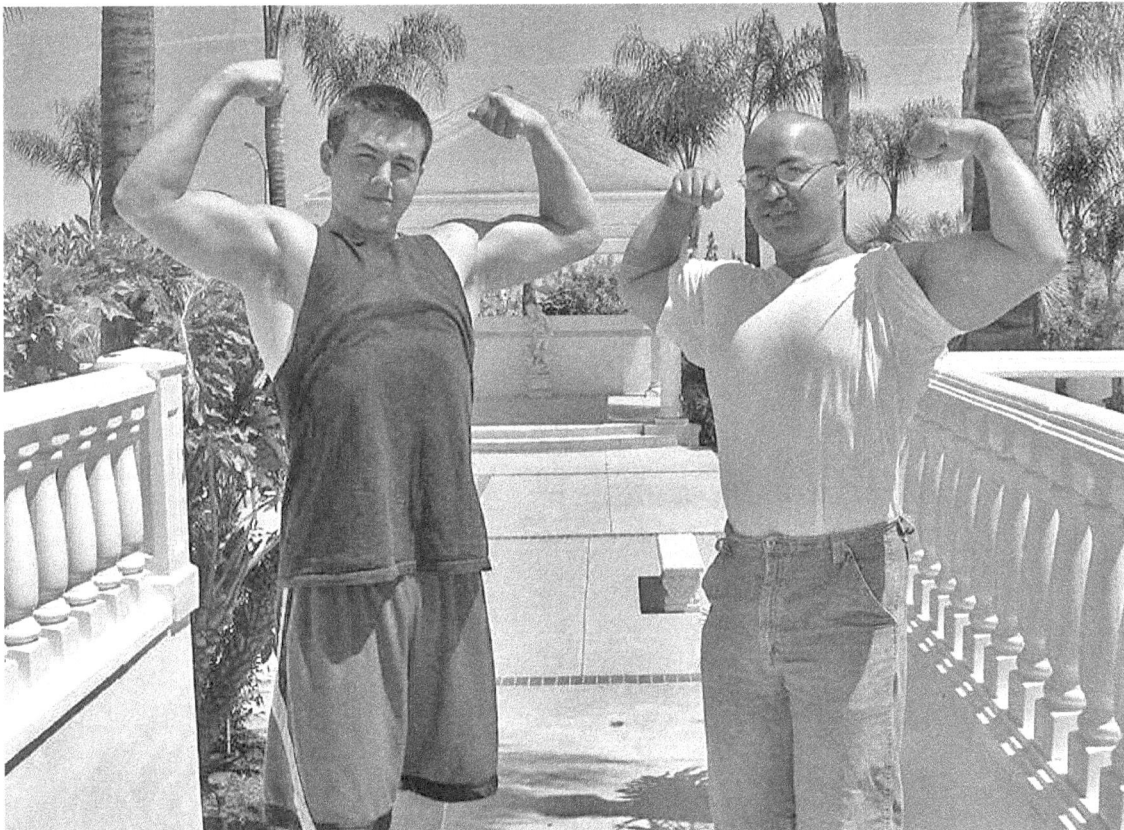

With Arthur Salas

CHAPTER 25

QUESTIONS AND ANSWERS

Over the span of 30 years as a person who worked out in gyms, and as a person who worked as a personal trainer, and through my personal websites, which I used to have up for almost 10 years, I received a number of questions and emails that made me think twice before answering and even made me do some research on. Many of these questions I remember very clearly and some I've saved in my file. I would like to share some of them with you because it might help you with your own questions in some ways.

This was from my own experience: I was once doing T-bar Rows and a friend of mine from the gym name Richard came up to me and asked me this question, *"How do you breathe during your exercises?"*

His question made me think about it for a moment and I certainly didn't have the correct answer at that time. I remember telling him, "I just leave my mouth open." After Richard said OK and went back to his training routine, unknowingly to him, he totally sabotaged my entire workout that day. I couldn't get back into the rhythm of it because I was too busy thinking about how to breathe during my exercises. Should I breathe in during my lifts or out, or maybe I should hold my breath so on and so forth.

There truly is a proper way to breathe during an intense set of your exercise. You take several large breaths before you begin your lift so this way you expand your lungs and get sufficient oxygen in. At the start of the lift you hold your breath for a second and once the weight is in a positive lift you breathe out till you have the weight at a peak contraction. Once you are at this position you take a deep breath again and start the negative part of your lift. During the negative lift you exhale and inhale continuously till you get to the extended position where you repeat the breathing cycle all over again.

Be very careful not to hold your breath during the positive lift. This can cause light headedness which it can sometimes lead to a black out. The heavier you go on the weights the more you are tempted in holding your breath throughout the positive lift. Always be in control of your breathing.

This question came to me via email from Tom in England: *"I've been doing H.I.T. for over 3 years now and I've seen some significant progress from it. But it seems of late that my progress has stopped completely and I haven't made any significant gains for quite some time now. My friend, who happened to be a personal trainer, suggest that I should go back to doing H.V.T. (High Volume Training) in order to shock and confuse my muscles and get them going again. I thought about going back to doing H.V.T. many times, but what do you think?"*

Well once the muscles are over that shock and confusion then what? This so-called shock and confusion is temporary for your body. It's more of a mental event rather than a physical one. Muscles respond by growing and getting stronger when they are stimulated sufficiently by H.I.T. H.V.T. is an overkill of that stimulation.

I understand completely why you would want to go back to doing H.V.T. Out of desperation you start to think that this is the solution to your plateau. I know because I, myself, experience plateaus all too often. I've gone back and forth between H.I.T. and H.V.T. only to find out later that I was wrong for doing this. I didn't make any progress at all. As a matter of fact according to my log I regressed.

Don't make the same mistake of training more and more frequently when you are in a plateau state. Instead examine if you are getting sufficient calories and nutrients from your diet. You might not be meeting the demands of your body. The bigger and the stronger you get the more your body will demand for calories and nutrients. Check and see if you are getting sufficient amount of sleep and rest. Also check how you are doing with your life's stress. If there are problems in these areas it can contribute to your plateau.

If none of these checks out then this may also be a sign that it is time to move to the next level of exercise. Meaning cutting back on the amount of exercises you do. If you are at the very advance stage already then I recommend that you take a week off every 6 to 8 weeks from training. Don't be afraid to take this occasional break from your workouts in order to better recuperate.

Edgar, I'm a female and I'm interested in becoming a competitive bodybuilder. How long must I train in order to get there?

If you train hard and are consistent with your clean diet you should be able to get ready for your first contest within 2 years or less. From my experience as a personal trainer I've seen young women, who train hard, develop much quicker than men. They are usually ready to compete within 14 to 16 month. It's because their muscles are not as large as the men. So this is why they have the potential to develop quicker.

I used to think that men would develop faster because of the level of hormones, particularly testosterone. But women who train at the same level of intensity as men can certainly develop quicker. Just that very few women are willing to engage themselves at that level of intensity.

When you do decide to enter don't expect anything big. Meaning, don't expect to be Ms. Universe any time soon. It takes time to mature in the Sport of Bodybuilding. Very few do well in their first or second year of competing, but definitely keep competing. This can be a great motivation for you to train harder in the gym and be more discipline with your diet and rest.

I recommend you compete no more than 2 times a year. Because preparing for the Sport of Bodybuilding can be really hard on the body. Since this is your first time, enter a local amateur contest first and take it from there.

I was born painfully thin and I remained so throughout my life. I truly believe it has something to do with my fast metabolism. Now that I'm 35 will I start to see any slowing down on my metabolism, so that I can start gaining some weight?

It depends. I used to work with a man who was in his 60's and weighed 150lbs. He had been at this weight ever since he was 18. But when I looked at his old pictures when he was a teenager and in his 20's it was clear that he was a lean and muscular 150lbs compared to what he was in his 60's where his muscles have atrophied and he was carrying more fat. So a slow down in metabolism doesn't always influence weight change. Yes metabolism does slow down as you age, but this is more due to the fact that your muscles are atrophying as you age and when this happen fat starts developing more easily, especially if you are still eating the same amount of food.

I take it though that you are doing weight training and you are frustrated in not gaining any weight. A slow down in your metabolism is not the answer for getting rid of your skinny self. It's meeting the demand of your metabolism and adding the plus calories to it that will help you.

For example if your body is burning 1800 calories a day to maintain itself and you are only eating 1500-1700 then you are not going to gain muscle weight. If you add 500 calories to that and start eating 2300 calories a day you will exceed the demand with enough calories to train hard and to develop your muscles.

How much does genetics play into this?

Quite a bit. Genetics determine what shape and size of our muscles, along with strength level, metabolism, and so forth. But the good thing is we all have the genetics to develop a strong and muscular body. Even though our genes determine the limitation of our development that limitation is often times never reached in our lifetime. I've been training for 30 years and I am almost 50 now, even though I am not making the same progress as I did when I started in my first 5 years it still surprises me to this day that I am able to gain some strength and mass here and there.

Me, personally, even though I don't have good genetics to become Mr. Universe, I am happy that I am no longer painfully thin. I don't compete in natural bodybuilding contest anymore; if I do decide to compete again it'll be just for the fun of it and not to win any major titles.

I want to know if it's OK to include single rep max lift to my H.I.T. workout?

I don't recommend single rep max lift for a couple of reasons. First, it is dangerous because you are going all out. If you are not properly warmed up the likeliness of an injury is great. Second, there's too much cheating involved in this lift. You may tend to arch your lower back too much if you are doing bench press and or bounce the weight off your chest just so you can do one rep. All these can lead to a potential injury. If you are doing barbell curls you may swing your body just to get that one rep max. Third, there's not enough stimulation to trigger your muscles to grow. Meaning not enough work into that one rep.

The least amount of reps I would recommend would be 4. At least with 4 reps you would have enough work to create stimulation to make your muscles grow, be safe from injuries, and to keep cheating out from your workouts. I know people like doing single rep max in order to find out how strong they are with a particular exercise. Even though I don't think this is the best way it really is up to you. Just be aware of what I've mentioned.

What do you think of Force Reps? I ask because my partner and I like to give each other 2-3 of this immediately after we hit positive failure. Will this help us develop more mass?

The stimulation is indeed greater with force reps, but it will take you a lot longer to recover from it. In other words, it's very easy to overtrain with force reps. You are better off to just hit positive failure till you can't move the weights any more, not even by an inch.

My training partner and I used to give each other force reps. After our workout both of us were too exhausted to do anything else throughout the day. All we wanted to do was sleep the day away. By the time we meet again for the next workout we were still sore and tired from the last workout.

Edgar, I was doing Lat Pulldowns the other day and I felt a strain on my right calf. I fear that I might have torn something. It was bad enough to make me stop working out. Believe it or not I went straight to the emergency room because I was worried. The doctor told me that I've strained my calf muscle and it wasn't a tear.

You did the right thing by going to the emergency room and had it checked right away. An injury is not something anyone should take lightly and think that they'll heal from it. There could be a tear that may require treatment.

Any time you engage in any physical activities there is a chance of getting injured. Even though you've taken all the precautionary steps like allowing yourself to fully recover, warming up sufficiently, and using good form there is still a chance of getting injured.

Once an injury has occurred go see a doctor right away. After doing this and you were sent home to recover I recommend you use a method that many fitness experts recommend, R.I.C.E.: Rest, Ice, Compress, and Elevate. You can also use R.I.C.E. before going to the doctor or if you are sure it's nothing serious and you want to treat it yourself. Now if your muscles feel tense after a workout I recommend you use a heating pad to help relax it.

Even though the guidelines I've provided in this book helps minimizes the chance for an injury. When it comes to working out it is not by any means a guarantee that you are going to be injury free. My word of advice, be sure to get a doctor's clearance that you are healthy enough to engage in strenuous exercises.

Absolutely! After I graduated from college one of the first jobs I had was working for an assisted living facility for the elderly, in the activities department. It made me sad when I saw many of the elderly there, who I think were healthy, using walkers, canes, and wheelchairs. Is not that there's something wrong with their legs, but it's because their leg muscles, as with the rest of their muscles, have atrophied so much that they weren't strong enough to give themselves adequate mobility.

Since I was working in the activities department it was my duty to schedule them for physical fitness activity. The facility would have a physical fitness instructor come almost on a daily basis and he or she would lead them in some sort of physical activities such chair aerobics, aqua aerobics, games such as passing the medicine ball around and chair yoga.

Although doing some kind of activity is better than not doing anything at all I became keenly aware how weight training would benefit them more than those activities. I truly believed back then they could regain some of the muscle mass they've lost over the years and improve their mobility. Along with that, they can also improve their bone density as well.

There are many fitness experts out there that would not recommend weight training for the elderly, especially not H.I.T., due to the fear that they might get hurt. If done properly, done on a machine instead of free weights, and if done in a H.I.T. fashion it is indeed quite safe. Yes, High Intensity Training you read it right, but with a slight twist: I would recommend that they lift the weights in an even slower manner, especially on the positive portion of the rep. They don't have to train to positive failure but at least get close to it. If they could do this 3 times a week I am sure they would regain some of the muscle mass, strength, and bone density they've lost.

I have bad reactions when I eat too much protein from meat, especially beef. I tend to feel nauseated and I get dizzy spells. Currently I'm eating very little protein. Will this hamper my progress?

Just as there are unique individuals out there who do not do very well in processing carbs in their system due to insulin there are indeed individuals who are even more unique because they do not process protein very well. My mother is one of them. Her joints tend to ache if she eats foods that are extremely high in protein. To this day the doctors haven't been able to give her a very good explanation as to why that is. But your concern as to whether or not this will affect your results. My answer to that is no.

Our bodies don't really need that much protein in order to support growth, maintenance, energy, and repair. If your concern about not meeting the minimum required amount then there is something else you can do. If eating meat is your problem then you can mix and match vegetables, grains, and wheat. Even though these have incomplete protein-mixing them up will give you a complete protein meal.

I have met and competed against natural bodybuilders who were pure vegetarians. They've successfully achieved their muscular bodies by learning which grains and vegetables to eat. Perhaps a vegetarian diet might be better for you. Try and see how your body does with this.

Is it alright to incorporate aerobics into my workouts?

If you are trying to get rid of your skinny self I would vote against it. Why would you want to do aerobics since you are already thin, but if your goal is to build muscles while trying to lose the fat or maintain your fat level to a minimum then it is alright. But keep this in mind, the more muscle mass you have the better your basal metabolic rate would be. This would make your body better at burning fat throughout the day and even in your sleep.

There are people out there and I too am one of them who enjoy doing aerobics. But you do have to be careful not to over do it. Remember your recovery ability should be left to building muscles and you must never allow aerobics to disturb that.

If you want aerobics to be a part of your training then what I would recommend you do low impact aerobics. Low impact aerobics are stationary cycling, walking, and such. I recommend you do 30 minutes a day 3 times a week or 20 minutes a day 4 times a week. Never do aerobics on the day you do your weight training.

If you feel exhausted after aerobics then you have over done it. If you feel a burning sensation on your legs due to lactic acid build up during aerobics then it is too intense. This would disturb your recovery ability. Of course if you are a beginner at this you will feel tired and a burning sensation in the beginning, but if this persist for more than 6 weeks then consider not doing it at all or at least wait till you get better developed with H.I.T.

I know there's more to physical activity than just weight training. I, myself, enjoy long distance cycling and hiking. I know some of you do as well. If you do plan on doing something like this then be sure to plan on taking a week off from weight training.

I don't get a whole lot of pump with H.I.T. compare to H.V.T. (High Volume Training).

The pump happens due to localized blood on the working muscle. You get more pump feeling from H.V.T. because you are doing set after set of the same exercise for the same muscle. With H.I.T. it is only one set taken to positive failure. There's not enough work there to cause blood congestion. Many people I've trained, including myself do get a pump feeling, but not to the same degree as one would get from H.V.T. Many times I don't get pumped at all.

A pumped feeling though is not a sure fire indicator that the muscle you are working on has been sufficiently stimulated to produce growth and strength. If the pump was all that's needed for gains then all we have to do is try and achieve that pump feeling at every workout and H.V.T. would be the sure bet.

A great degree of pump is mostly achieved by using light to medium heavy weights where the rep range are anywhere from 10-12. We know by lifting weights that is heavy to you and taking it to positive failure forces your muscles to adapt to that high degree of resistance. Light and medium heavy weights do not give the same result. Sure you'll improve your appearance and your fitness level, but if you are looking for muscle density and increase in strength then H.I.T. is the way to go.

Edgar, I'm in my early 20's and I have a problem gaining muscles. No matter how much food I eat or how hard I train I still can't put on the muscles I want. Could it be that I have low testosterone? I'm thinking about taking steroids.

Ah…I had similar thoughts back then when I was in my early 20's. One of the gym members suggested that I take steroids to help me bulk up. I decided against it because I wanted to keep my health and to not have any future health problems. It wasn't till I discovered H.I.T. and paying more attention to my calorie intake I started gaining muscle weight did I realize that I didn't have a problem at all with my testosterone.

But there are some men out there that do suffer from low testosterone levels in their body. The best thing you should do is to have your testosterone check by a doctor. If you do have low testosterone then let the doctor prescribe it. Don't just blindly go to a black market and buy yourself testosterone or steroids. Chances are you might not know what you're doing.

But first I want you to try H.I.T., if you haven't tried it, and see if this will help you gain muscles. Start counting your daily calories. You can checkout a Food Calorie Index book at a local library and get a rough estimation as to how many calories you are eating a day. Once you know how many calories there are then add 500 more calories. You can do this by adding a meal or a protein meal.

When doing weight training is it better to have a training partner?

There are a lot of advantages to having a training partner. For one thing they can certainly push you during your workouts and you can certainly get more motivation from them as well. Just be sure to have a training partner who is willing to push it hard in the gym as you do.

I was very fortunate and bless to have my late wife, Adriana Garcia, as my training partner. Back then I didn't think she would make a good training partner because of her lack of experience and knowledge in weight training, but she cared a lot for my progress and she pushed me hard – harder than any training partners I've had in the past.

Adriana watched my form to make sure I wasn't getting sloppy. She counted my reps and she made sure my reps were done in proper rep scheme. And just when I thought I hit positive failure with my exercise she would force me to try for another rep. Nowadays I train by myself, because sadly Adriana is gone, but I can still hear her pushing me hard in the gym. So my intensity in the gym hasn't changed one bit.

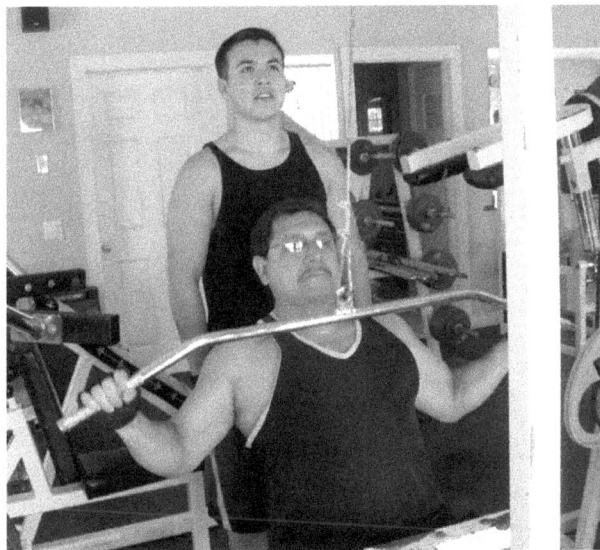

Jorge Sanchez has his grandson, Arthur Salas, for his training partner.

197

"It ain't about how hard you hit. It's about how hard you can get hit and keep moving forward. It's how much you can take and keep moving forward. That's how winning is done!"

--Rocky Balboa

PART IX

Importance of Psychology

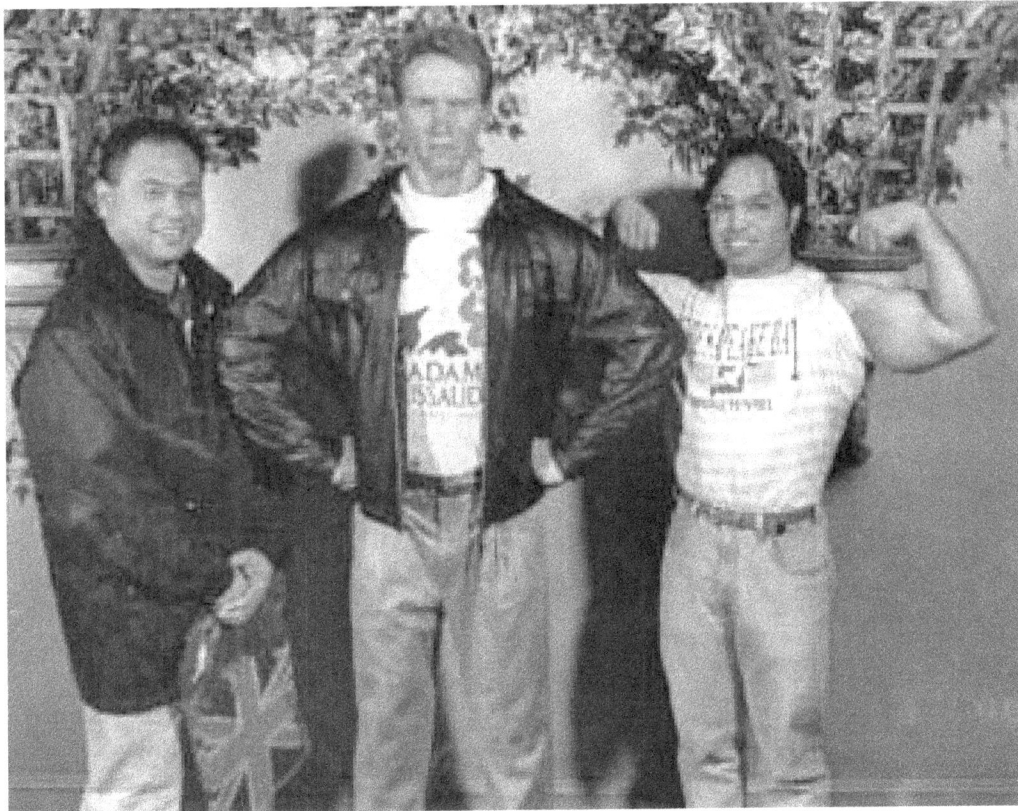

My brother, Edwin, and I with a wax figure of Arnold Schwarzenegger

CHAPTER 26

THE IMPORTANCE OF PSYCHOLOGY

I can tell you how to workout, eat properly, and get sufficient amount of rest, but if you are not mentally into it your progress would be a fiasco. Psychology is very important when it comes to getting rid of your skinny self. It would make or break you. To simply put it, you have to believe in yourself. Your body is willing only if your mind is.

In the beginning I was very much intimidated in going to a gym because I was very much self consciously aware of my skinny state and I was too embarrass to see myself or to be seen working out with the guys at Mt. Olympus Gym who were twice my size. But I was fortunate to have friends like Denny Kakos, the gym owner, who pushed me to train hard. In a couple of years I was one of the strongest and the biggest guy in his gym. It is that mental drive that made me train hard in order to reach my goal. I like to think nobody trained harder at Mt. Olympus Gym than me.

At Mr. Olympus Gym I met a man there by the name of Steve who used to workout along side with some of the professional bodybuilders from the Golden Era, 1970's at Gold's Gym.

He once told me that the famous Arnold Schwarzenegger would come back to train at Gold's Gym after taking a long vacation from Austria. He would be training for the upcoming Mr. Olympia contest. He mentioned to me how Arnold would look half the size as he was from his best condition after coming back from Austria, but in a couple of months or so of training he would looked incredible again and ready for the Mr. Olympia show.

The main thing Steve told me was how focused and motivated Arnold was when he trained. He said to me if a bomb goes off outside the gym, Arnold wouldn't get distracted by it, because he was that focus on his training. He said when Arnold would come into the gym the whole atmosphere would change and the energy level would change. Everyone would train harder because of his presence.

Focus on Yourself

I have received a couple of emails from men and women all over the world asking me how to deal with the feeling of intimidation in the gym. I always tell them to focus on themselves.

Often times we get out of focus in the gym because we pay too much attention to the people around us. We look at what others are doing and we look to see or wonder if others are looking at us. When we do this we really get too self conscious of ourselves.

Focus on yourself only. It shouldn't matter what others are doing in the gym or if they are looking at you or not. Focus on your workout and try to get through it with the best of your effort. If your mind is not focused on your workout then it won't be fruitful. Remember, your body is only willing if your mind is really into it.

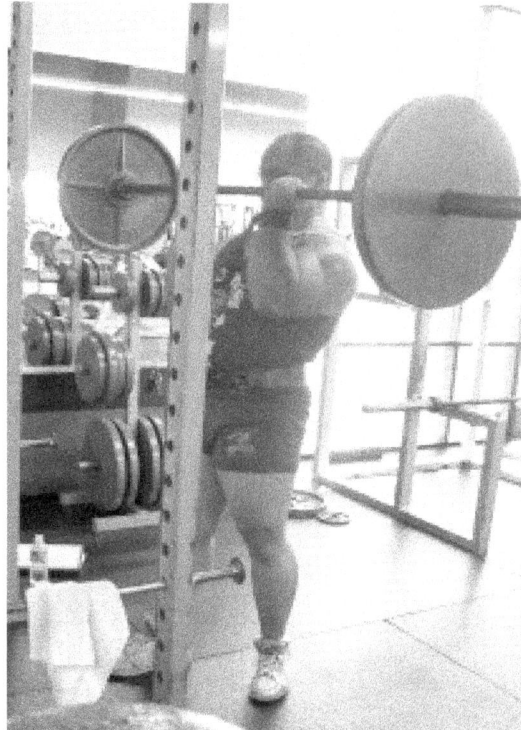

Without focusing on myself I wouldn't be able to lift this much weight.

Leave It Outside the Gym

I recall training this lady who had just broken up with her boyfriend of 4 years. I spent 50 minutes listening to her ranting about him. When she finally decided to start her workout I still continued listening to her rant during her workout session with me. She even did this while in the middle of her working set. By the end of her workout session she didn't get a good workout at all and even she mentioned it to me. It would've been better for her to have never worked out and dealt with her emotions first before coming to the gym.

We are all faced with certain problems in our lives, but to take it in the gym would spell disaster. You can't expect yourself to have a good workout if you keep thinking about your problems. The gym should be a haven for you to unwind, relax mentally, and train hard. If you can do this without thinking about your problems outside the gym and you get through your workout you'll find that you actually feel better about yourself. You will, more likely, leave the gym with a clear mind. And with a clear mind you might perhaps deal with your problems in a better way.

Get Psycho

When I start my workout I really get in the zone. I see myself as a ball of energy waiting to unleash on all my exercises. I don't really care about the atmosphere in the gym because I create my own. I don't really care if people are looking at me or if I'm being too loud with my grunts. My main thing is accomplishing my goal with my exercises.

It should be that way with you. Go in the gym totally focused, feeling energetic, and totally motivated in accomplishing your goals. If you have a training partner push each other to do more reps and to work hard. Pat each other on the back and say positive things about each other's workout. Most importantly, be sure to have fun with it.

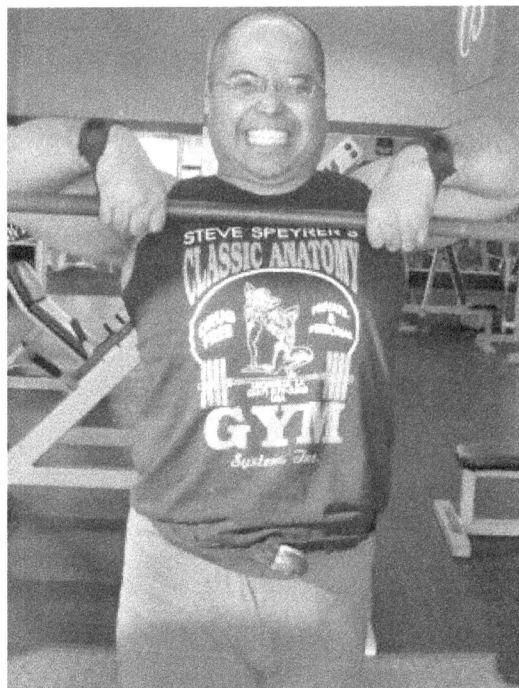

Get psyched up with your workout.

Visualize

Before I even start my exercises in my mind's eye I've already done them. I already saw myself doing a rep or two more than before on each of my exercises' target rep. Visualization is very important in your workout. To be able to see yourself pushing hard on the exercises and to see yourself accomplishing and surpassing your target rep will help you achieve your goal.

I remember my training partner, Jim Herman. He was used to doing 80lbs of dumbbell presses for his chest. For a couple of months he was stuck on using this weight for 8 reps and he couldn't move up from it. I told him to visualize himself doing the exercise and doing more reps before engaging in it.

After doing this and psyching himself up almost to a point of insanity I handed him the dumbbells and he did presses with it. He was very disappointed after finishing his set because he couldn't out do his personal best of 8 reps. But when I told him that he did 8 reps with 90lbs instead of 80lbs he was quite shock.

So visualize yourself accomplishing your goal. Before you even touch the weight visualize yourself already lifting it and doing more than what you expected. Also use this tool to see how you want to look like. See in your mind's eye your muscles growing. This visualization technique would indeed give you a better mind and body connection.

Be Proud of Yourself

Every time you finish your workout in the gym you should see it as an accomplishment that you can be proud of. Because it is a step towards in getting rid of your skinny self. Every time you see a pound of gain on your weight scale or an increase in the weights you use on your exercises you know that you are moving forward and that is something you should always be proud of. Progress is all about moving forward.

I mentioned earlier how important it is to set short term goals and long term goals. Short term goals are goals that are achievable at a certain short amount of time. Each time you accomplish one of your short term goals it is a step toward your long term goal. Until finally, you break that long term goal. So be proud of your accomplishments even if they are small like finishing your workout in the gym and breaking one of your short term goals. In the end you will reap the benefit from this.

Go For It!

You now have the knowledge as to what it takes to get rid of your skinny self. The rest is all about application. It truly is up to you. ***Go for it!***

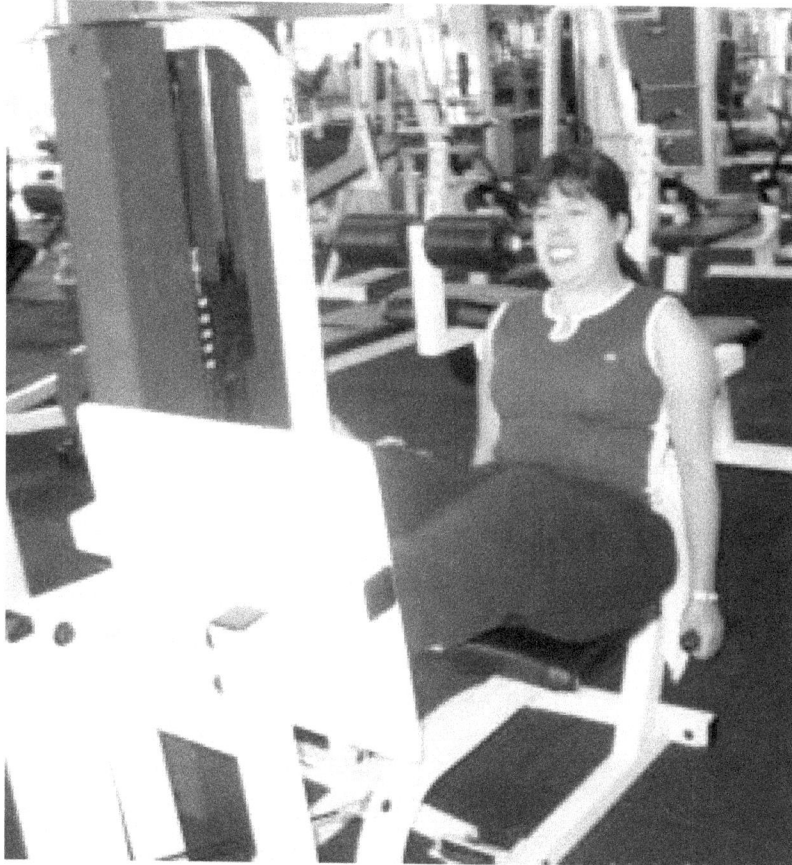

Adriana Garcia

FINISH

In Loving Memory of *Adriana Rocio Garcia*

1972-2011

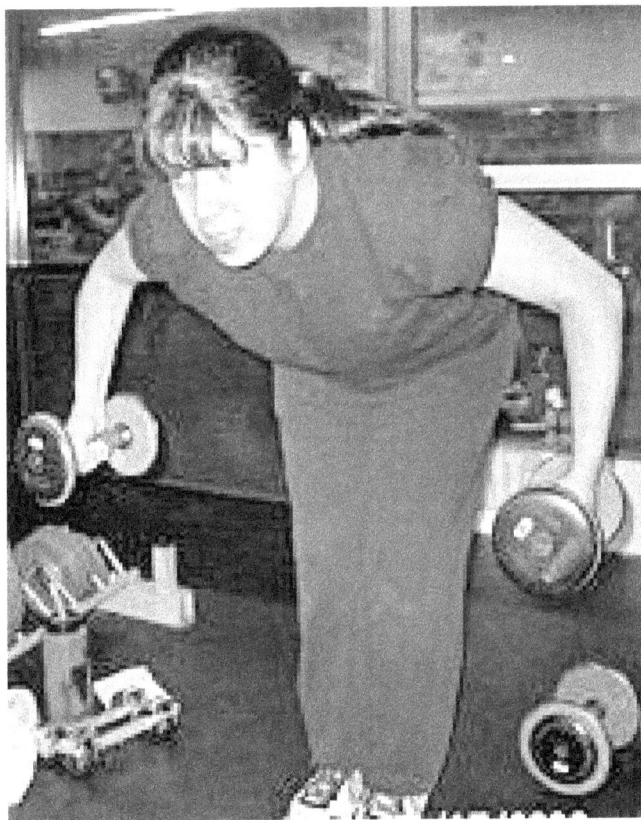

www.ingramcontent.com/pod-product-compliance
Lightning Source LLC
Chambersburg PA
CBHW080048280326

41934CB00014B/3253